The Simple Guide to Having a Baby

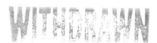

of Parent Trust for Washington Children;
authors of *Pregnancy, Childbirth, and the Newborn*

Meadowbrook Press
distributed by Simon & Schuster
New York, NY

Library of Congress Cataloging-in-Publication Data

Names: Whalley, Janet, 1945- author.
Title: The simple guide to having a baby / Janet Whalley [and three others].
Description: Third edition. | Minnetonka : Meadowbrook Press ; New York : Distributed by Simon &
    Schuster, [2016] | Revision of: Simple guide to having a baby / by Janet Whalley ... [et al.]. c2012.
Identifiers: LCCN 2016014242 (print) | LCCN 2016023005 (ebook) | ISBN 9781501112713 (paperback) |
    ISBN 9780881665741 (meadowbrook press) | ISBN 9781451670790 (ebook)
Subjects: LCSH: Pregnancy--Popular works. | Childbirth--Popular works. | Newborn infants--
    Care--Popular works. | BISAC: HEALTH & FITNESS / Pregnancy & Childbirth. | MEDICAL /
    Gynecology & Obstetrics. | FAMILY & RELATIONSHIPS / Parenting / Motherhood.
Classification: LCC RG525 .S587 2016 (print) | LCC RG525 (ebook) | DDC 618.2--dc23
LC record available at https://lccn.loc.gov/2016014242

Editor: Heidi Hogg
Creative Director: Tamara JM Peterson
Index: Beverlee Day
Cover photo: © Getty Images
Text: © 2016, 2011, 2005 by Parent Trust for Washington Children
The illustrations in this book were developed by Susan Spellman © 2005, 2010
The line drawings were created by Shanna dela Cruz, © 1994–2010 Ruth Ancheta

Although the authors and publisher have made every effort to ensure that the information in this book is
accurate and current, only your caregiver knows you and your health history well enough to make specific
recommendations. The authors, editors, and publisher disclaim any liability from the use of this book.

Published by:
Meadowbrook Press
6110 Blue Circle Drive, Suite 237
Minnetonka, Minnesota, 554343
www.MeadowbrookPress.com

BOOK TRADE DISTRIBUTION by:
Simon and Schuster
a division of Simon and Schuster, Inc.
1230 Avenue of the Americas
New York, New York, 10020

22 21 20 19 18 17 16   10 9 8 7 6 5 4 3 2

Printed in the United States of America

Dedication

To the thousands of new and expectant parents
we've worked with over the years and to our families,
who have taught us about birth and being parents.

To our husbands and to our children and their families:

Peter Simkin
Andy, Bess, Alfred, Arshia, Charlie, Eva Rose, and Jonathan
Linny, Peter, and Callie
Mary, Greg, Sara Jane, and Amelia
Elizabeth and Cole

Doug Whalley
Scott, Heidi, Kate, and Adelyn
Mike, Leslie, and Finn

Jerry Keppler
Eric, Courtney, Lucas, and Noah
Heidi and Paul

Peter Durham
Martin, Izzi, and Ben

Thank You

We wish to thank our editors: Joseph Gredler, Megan McGinnis, Christine Zuchora-Walske, and Alicia Ester, who helped with previous editions of this book, and Heidi Hogg, who helped with this edition.

We want to thank the following people for their assistance with reading and giving feedback on the first edition of this book: Katie Ladner, Lauren Valk Lawson, Creagh Miller, and Tera Schreiber.

For drawings and design of this book, we wish to thank: Tamara JM Peterson, Susan Spellman, and Ruth Ancheta.

For help and support, we thank the staff of Parent Trust for Washington Children and its Great Starts program, which has been helping new families since 1950.

Contents

Introduction

We wrote *The Simple Guide to Having a Baby* to help you understand what happens during pregnancy, birth, and the weeks after having your baby. We want to help you do these three things:

1. Have a healthy and comfortable pregnancy. There are so many things you can do to help make pregnancy more enjoyable and less stressful.
2. Plan and prepare for childbirth. Learning what to expect, practicing coping skills, and knowing important questions to ask will help you have a safe and satisfying birth experience.
3. Learn how to care for a baby and get parenting off to a great start. You'll know the basics of newborn care and feeding, and know about resources for learning more as your child grows.

Wishing you a wonderful pregnancy, a happy birth day, and joyful parenting,

Janet Whalley, Penny Simkin,
Ann Keppler, and Janelle Durham

Reading This Book

This guide is intended to be quicker and easier to read than others available to pregnant women. If you want more in-depth information, please read our book *Pregnancy, Childbirth, and the Newborn: The Complete Guide.*

To understand new words or medical terms: Look in the glossary on pages 181–189.

To find more information on a topic within this book: When a topic is discussed in more than one section of the book, we include the other page numbers to help you find it (for example, "see pages 23-25"). You can also look in the index on pages 190-195.

To find more information outside this book: We've included links to online resources in the chapters. In the section called Help for You and Your Baby on pages 175-180, we give contact information for agencies that provide helpful services for new parents.

CHAPTER 1
Preparing for Pregnancy

Before you get pregnant, think about whether you're emotionally and physically ready. This chapter will help you explore your feelings and learn how a healthy lifestyle can help your body get ready to carry a baby. It's best if you begin preparing for pregnancy at least 4 months before you *conceive* (become pregnant), but even if you're trying to get pregnant right now, you can improve your chances and learn how to have a healthy pregnancy with the tips found here.

Note

If you're already pregnant, you can skip this chapter. Don't worry if you didn't prepare beforehand. Just start making healthy choices today. And remember this chapter for future pregnancy planning.

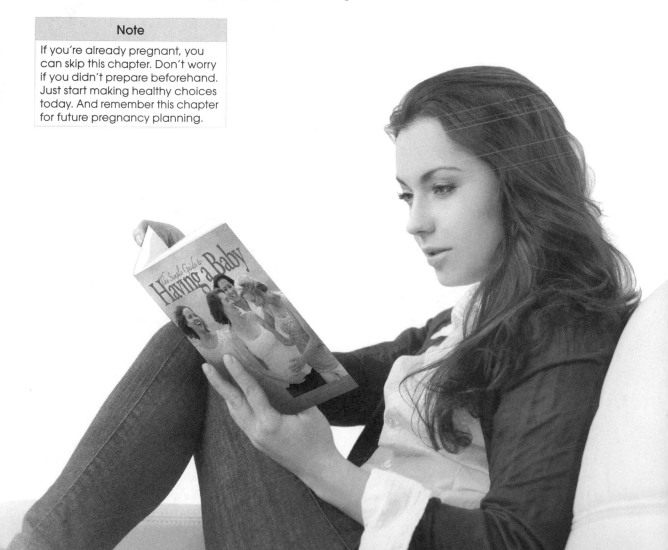

Note to Future Fathers and Co-parents

It's helpful for you to read this chapter and be sure you're ready for a baby too. Becoming a parent is a major lifestyle change for both partners. Fathers-to-be can also focus on becoming healthier before conceiving, because healthy sperm will help create a healthy baby. Try to reach a healthy weight and try to avoid or reduce alcohol, smoking, illegal drugs, and harmful chemicals. Your weight and these substances can reduce your sperm count or activity (making it harder to start a pregnancy) or cause problems with your sperm that can affect the baby's health. Learn more at http://www.cdc.gov/preconception/men.html.

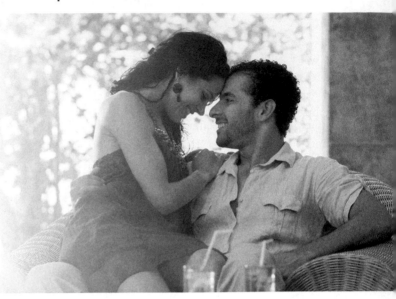

Are You Ready for a Baby? Questions to Explore

Before you get pregnant, you and your partner may want to consider the following questions. You don't need to have all the answers or have all the "right" answers, but the more prepared you are, the easier parenting may be. (*Note*: If you plan to be a single parent, some questions won't apply to you. But you may want to think about how your network of friends and family may or may not support you.)

- **Your interest in raising a child:** Do you like being around children? Would you enjoy being a parent? Do you like doing kid activities? Are you patient enough to deal with the noise, chaos, and responsibility?
- **Your partner's interest in raising a child:** Are you and your partner equally committed to becoming parents?
- **Health of your relationship:** Do you love and trust each other? Do you fight a lot? If you don't get along now, it will be even harder when you have a baby. Learn ways to work out conflicts before getting pregnant.
- **Family values:** Do you have similar ideas about parenting? Do you agree on how you spend your time and money? If you have different religious beliefs, have you discussed how you'll handle them?
- **Support and community:** How well do you get along with your own parents? Do you have friends or family who would support you with parenting? Are there good resources for parents in your community?
- **Health and lifestyle:** Are you and your partner both in good physical health? Are there any lifestyle changes you can make to better your chances of a healthy pregnancy (such as exercising or giving up smoking)? Are you ready to give up the freedom to do what you want when you want?

- **Finances:** What will your income be after having a baby? Have you considered expenses such as diapers, baby clothes and equipment, and child care? Does your insurance cover maternity care and birth? (Learn more about insurance at http://www.healthcare.gov.) Will you be able to take time off from work?
- **Career goals:** How will having a baby affect your career? Could you handle a child and a job or school at the same time? Will having a child at this time keep you from reaching your goals? If so, would you resent it?
- **Your reasons for having a baby:** What are your reasons for wanting a baby? There are many good reasons to start a family. However, there are also wrong reasons: because everyone else is doing it, because you hope it will fix your relationship, or because you just want someone to love you. People who choose parenthood for the wrong reasons often regret it in the future.

As you discuss your answers to these questions, you will begin to get a picture of whether now is the right time for you to have a baby. If you feel comfortable with your answers, you're probably ready for parenthood. If you have concerns, think about whether they will go away if you wait awhile or change something.

Cami's Story

During my 20s and 30s, I was in and out of a few long-term relationships. With each partner, I had long conversations about kids. I knew I really wanted a baby someday. But it was never the right time: either our finances weren't good, or it was a busy time at work, or our relationship wasn't that great. Looking back now, I'm glad I decided not to have a baby each of those times.

Then I met Chris, and finally I feel like I'm in the right place and with the right person. We're looking forward to starting a family together.

Is It Time for Another Baby?

If you already have one or more older children, here are some things to think about and discuss with your partner or support team:

- **How long has it been since your last birth?** For the healthiest pregnancy and baby, it's best to wait at least 18 months before starting again. Starting a pregnancy in the first year after a birth increases the chance of preterm birth, low birth weight, and health problems for you.
- **Are you ready to care for another child?** Ask other parents how far apart their children are in age, what's been easy or hard about parenting two or more children, and what they recommend. What works for you may be different than what works for them, but it helps to know ahead of time what other people have experienced.

Get Fit and Healthy

Once you decide you're ready for a baby, it's time to evaluate your health. The healthier you are before pregnancy, the easier your pregnancy and birth will be and the healthier your baby will be. We'll give you lots of tips in this chapter. If you want to learn more about healthy pregnancy, we recommend checking out www.marchofdimes.org.

Eat a Healthy Diet

Choose healthy, whole foods (organically grown, if possible) and make sure you get at least 400 micrograms of folic acid every day (4–5 milligrams a day if you have diabetes or epilepsy, or are obese). Folic acid lowers the risk of *miscarriage* (death of a baby in early pregnancy) and some birth defects. Foods such as bread and cereal often have added folic acid, or you can take folic acid as a pill. If it's affordable, take a prenatal vitamin or other multivitamin. They're a good way to get folic acid and all of your nutrients.

To learn more about healthy eating, read chapter 4. The foods that will be good for you in pregnancy are good for you before pregnancy. (But don't add any extra calories yet.)

Drink Plenty of Healthy Liquids

Drink 64 to 96 ounces (8 to 12 cups) of liquid a day. Water is the best choice. Juice and soda have a lot of added sugar, and many sodas contain caffeine. Caffeine can make conceiving harder.

Get to a Healthy Weight

It will be easier to get pregnant if you're at a healthy weight. Both underweight and overweight people can have trouble conceiving, and they have a higher chance of miscarriage and premature birth once pregnant. If the father-to-be is underweight or obese, it affects his sperm and may make it harder to conceive a pregnancy.

Do what you can to reach a healthy weight before becoming pregnant. Being overweight also increases your risk of getting diabetes or high blood pressure during pregnancy or needing a cesarean birth. If you're heavy, your baby is more likely to be big at birth, have birth defects, and be overweight as he gets older.

If you've had an eating disorder, work with a counselor and your doctor to prepare for pregnancy.

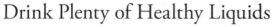

Maria's Story

After we got married, we knew that we wanted to have a baby in the next year or so. We wanted to have a healthy baby, so I scheduled a checkup with my doctor. I got caught up on my shots. I learned what to eat and what to avoid. We were really happy to learn that most of the foods we liked were good for me. I would have hated it if I had to stop eating spicy foods. My doctor did suggest that I try to add some exercise. My sister was really heavy when she wanted a baby. It made it harder for her to get pregnant, and she had gestational diabetes during pregnancy.

Exercise

For both the mother- and father-to-be, moderate exercise (2 to 7 hours per week) can increase your chances of getting pregnant. You'll have an easier time handling the physical changes of pregnancy if you're strong and fit. Exercise also improves your mood and lowers stress.

See Your Dentist for a Checkup

Your dental health can affect the health of your whole body, so have a dental checkup. Have any cavities fixed, but ask for fillings without mercury. Treat any gum disease because infections can cause problems during pregnancy. If you don't have dental insurance, go to http://www.freedentalcare.us to search for low-cost dental care.

See Your Medical Doctor for a Checkup

You and the baby's father will both want to see a doctor for a full checkup. He or she will screen you for sexually transmitted infections, which can make getting pregnant tougher and can cause miscarriage or birth defects for your baby.

Talk to your doctor about any medications you're taking. You'll want to avoid *anticoagulants* (blood thinners), such as warfarin (Coumadin); oral steroids for asthma; the acne medication isotretinoin (Accutane); the ulcer medication misoprostol (Cytotec); and oral birth control pills and the birth control shot (Depo-Provera). If you're prescribed any new medications, make sure your doctor and pharmacist know you're planning to get pregnant.

If you have any chronic (long-lasting) health problems, work with your doctor to manage them. They can harm you and your baby if not well controlled before pregnancy. Here are some tips:

- **Diabetes:** Improve your diet and exercise. Use medication wisely to keep your blood sugar in control. Ask your doctor if you need to change from oral medication to insulin.
- **High blood pressure (hypertension):** Improve your blood pressure by eating better, exercising, and quitting tobacco use. Work with your doctor to adjust your medications, as some are harmful to babies.
- **Epilepsy:** Take 4–5 milligrams of folic acid daily. Adjust medications as needed to best control your seizures. Most seizure medications increase the chance of birth defects. Work with your doctor to find the one that works best for you with the least risks.
- **Depression/anxiety:** Seek counseling and support before, during, and after your pregnancy. Ask your doctor or pharmacist about medications. Some are okay for pregnancy. If you have mild depression or anxiety, consider stopping medication for pregnancy. However, if you have bipolar disorder, severe depression, or anxiety, it is probably best to keep taking your medication.
- **Hypothyroid and hyperthyroid:** Before conception, be sure your thyroid levels are stable. Talk to your doctor about adjusting your medication in early pregnancy.

Get Up-to-Date on Your Vaccinations

If you haven't had chicken pox, you should get the varicella vaccine. If you're not immune to rubella (German measles), get the rubella or MMR vaccine. If you're at risk of sexually transmitted or blood exposure, ask your doctor about getting the hepatitis B vaccine. Wait 1–3 months after getting vaccinated before you conceive.

These vaccines are important to protect against these illnesses. If a baby is exposed to them during pregnancy or birth, they can cause miscarriage, birth defects, or lifelong health problems.

Ask Your Doctor about Genetic Screening

Some diseases are more common for people of certain ethnic backgrounds. (For example, African Americans are more at risk for sickle cell anemia.) It's possible that you or your partner could be a

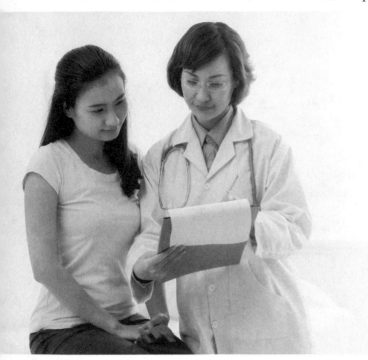

carrier (someone who can pass on a disease) even if you don't have the disease yourself. If members of your family have a certain disease, there's a higher chance your baby will too. Your doctor may recommend a *screening* (test to find out if you are a carrier). A genetic counselor can help you understand the results. Some people, after learning about a risk, choose not to become pregnant. Others will make plans during pregnancy so they can care for their baby's special health challenges.

For more information about genetic screening and preconception health care, visit "Pregnancy: Preconception Health" at the website for the Office on Women's Health, http://www.womens health.gov/pregnancy/before-you-get -pregnant/preconception-health.html.

Limit Preconception Hazards

Before you become pregnant, try to stay away from things that could harm your health.

Avoid Harmful Substances

Alcohol, tobacco, and street drugs are substances that can seriously harm a pregnancy. Caffeine can also have negative effects. Both you and the father-to-be should try to avoid these for 4 months before you plan to get pregnant. If you can't quit them completely, then use them less often. The less you use, the healthier it will be for you and the baby.

			Effect of Drugs on Pregnancy		
	Makes sperm less healthy	Make it harder to get pregnant	Increases miscarriage risk	Increases risk of birth defects	Increases risk of premature birth
Caffeine*	X	X	X		
Alcohol	X	X?	X	X	X
Tobacco	X	X	X	X	X
Street drugs	X	X	X	X	X
*Drinking 1–2 cups (8–16 ounces) of coffee or soda each day is okay. But consuming more than that, or using energy drinks or other products with a lot of caffeine, is a bad idea.					

For more on harmful substances and resources to help you quit using them, see chapter 4 or visit the Planning Pregnancy pages on http://www.childbirthconnection.org.

Be Careful about Environmental Hazards

Both you and the father-to-be should try to avoid being around the following, which are linked to infertility, miscarriage, and birth defects:

- **Lead:** Stay away from traffic fumes and be careful if remodeling a home that might have lead-based paint or lead pipes.
- **Mercury:** Don't eat fish containing high levels of mercury. (See http://www.nrdc.org/health/effects /mercury/guide.asp for a list of unsafe fish.) Don't get a new tattoo or tooth fillings with mercury.
- **Aluminum:** Avoid food or beverages cooked or stored in aluminum, and use aluminum-free baking powder, antacids, and deodorant.
- **Other hazardous chemicals and substances (solvents, pesticides, chemical fumes from paints, thinners, wood preservatives, glues, benzene, dry cleaning fluids, carbon monoxide, anesthetic gases, X-rays and radioactive materials):** Both mothers-to-be and fathers-to-be should try to avoid or reduce use.
- **Bisphenol A (BPA) plastics and phthalates:** Try to avoid plastic containers with the numbers 3 or 7 or the letters PC on the bottom. Don't microwave food in plastic containers. Limit the use of canned food, as can linings may include BPA.
- **High temperatures:** Before pregnancy, dads-to-be should limit saunas and hot tub use to fewer than 10 minutes and keep the temperature under 102°F. If his testicles get too hot, he will make less sperm. (You should avoid high temperatures once pregnant. See page 45 for more information.)

If you're exposed to hazards at work, shower afterward. Wash your work clothes separately. Ask your employer for Material Safety Data Sheets (MSDS), fresh air, and protective gear.

Prevent Infections

Wash your hands often. Use gloves when cleaning, when caring for others who might be sick, and when cleaning a cat's litter box. Use good food-safety practices to protect from food poisoning. Cook all meats completely. Keep foods that might spoil in the refrigerator.

Get Emotionally Ready

When you're planning for a baby, it's just as important to be emotionally healthy as it is to be physically healthy.

Focus on Your Feelings

Many people have had difficult life experiences that lead to feelings of sadness, fear, or anger. These feelings can make coping with the challenges of pregnancy, labor, and parenting harder. Explore your feelings and come to terms with your experiences before you get pregnant. See a counselor, attend a support group, read self-help books, or find supportive friends. These steps will help you learn new coping skills.

Reduce Stress

Stress can raise your blood pressure and make you sick. It can also lead to poor eating and sleep habits, and increase your risk of miscarriage or premature birth. Try to reduce the stress in your life before pregnancy. Take these steps:

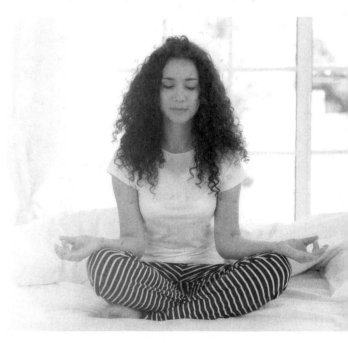

- Figure out what causes you stress. What places, people, activities, or demands are hard to handle?
- Avoid those stressful things, if you can. Find ways to cope with the things you can't avoid. Ask for help.
- Get your feelings out instead of holding them inside. Talk to a friend or a counselor, make art, or write in a journal.
- Do things that help you feel good. Exercise, sleep well, eat well, spend time with friends, and do other things that you enjoy.

Work on Your Relationship with Your Partner

If you and your partner have a strong, positive relationship now, your relationship may grow stronger as you parent together. But if your relationship is not good now, the stress of pregnancy and parenting will probably make things worse for you as a couple.

Talk with your partner about what's going well and what you don't like. Work together on making the relationship better. You may want to meet with a counselor, read a book about relationships and parenting (such as *And Baby Makes Three* by John Gottman and Julie Schwartz Gottman), or go to a workshop on relationships.

Find Support for Single Parenting

If you will be parenting on your own, make sure you have a good support network of friends and family. Search online for a local support group for single parents.

Fertility Issues

If it's taking longer to get pregnant than you'd hoped, keep the following information in mind:

- It's *normal* to take 6 months to conceive. If you're over 35, it may take even longer.
- Timing is important. You *ovulate* (release an egg) about 14 days before your period (if your cycle is 28 days long, this would be on the fourteenth day, but if your cycle is 33 days, this would be on the nineteenth day). If you have sex in the 3 days before ovulation or on the day you ovulate, you're more likely to get pregnant.
- In general, there's no need to have medical care for fertility issues unless you've been trying for more than a year. (If you're over age 40, get help after 6 months.)
- *Infertility* (having a hard time starting a pregnancy) is often due to an imbalance that can be fixed. Exercise, pay attention to your diet, and avoid hazards. Eating certain nutrients, taking herbal supplements, and acupuncture can all be helpful.

If you want to learn about ways to improve your fertility, download our free e-book on preconception, available on iTunes and Amazon. If these tips don't help, consider using assisted reproductive technology (ART). To learn more, visit http://www.cdc.gov/art/index.html.

Tanya's Story

With my first pregnancy, it took 4 or 5 months of trying to get pregnant. I now know it's normal, but back then I worried that it would never happen. This time, I made sure to take good care of myself, and I learned things Jason and I could do to boost my chances of getting pregnant.

I wanted my kids to be about three years apart, but I also really wanted the baby to be born in the summer, so my mom could help out (she's a teacher). I used all the ideas I could find about monitoring my cycles and timing when we had sex. Luckily, I got pregnant only a month after we started trying!

Conclusion

This chapter suggests many things you can do to increase your chances of getting pregnant soon and having the healthiest pregnancy possible. But don't feel like you have to do all these things or make everything perfect before you start on the path toward parenthood. One of the first lessons of parenting is to be proud of yourself for the good choices you make and to go easy on yourself for any mistakes you make. Just do the best you can each day.

CHAPTER 2

Now That
You're Pregnant

Pregnancy is a time of wonder. You wonder what you'll feel like later in your pregnancy. You wonder how your baby grows. You may also wonder about birth and how it'll feel to become a parent. This section describes what's happening during pregnancy. Read on to learn more about these topics:

- how your body changes
- how you may feel during pregnancy
- how your baby develops

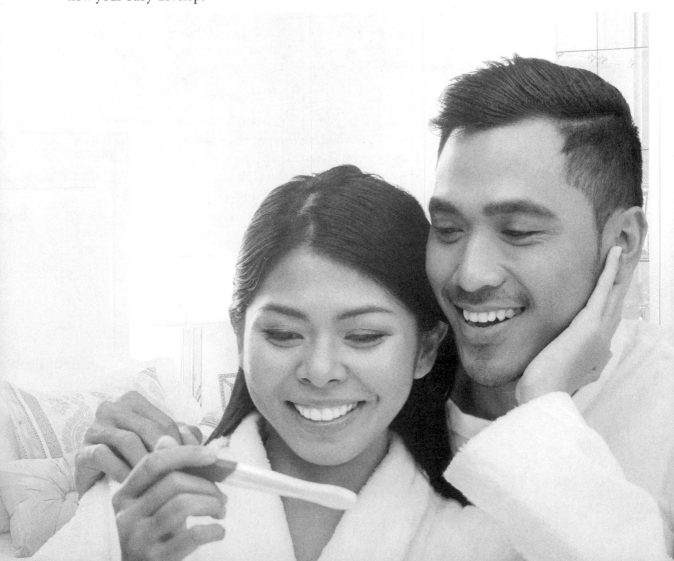

Becoming Pregnant

A woman can become pregnant by having sexual intercourse around the time of the month her *ovary* (sex gland inside her belly) releases an egg. When a man's semen goes into her vagina, his *sperm cells* (from his sex glands called *testicles*) travel toward her egg. When 1 sperm cell enters her egg, she becomes pregnant.

We'll start this chapter with a quick review of words that your doctor or midwife may use at visits during your pregnancy.

- The unborn baby is called a *fetus.*
- The *placenta* is an organ you grow during pregnancy to support the developing baby.
- The placenta makes *hormones* (substances that tell your body to make changes that are needed to grow a baby). These hormones (estrogen, progesterone, and others) affect how you feel both physically and emotionally.
- The *umbilical cord* connects the placenta to your baby. It carries food nutrients and oxygen to your baby and takes away waste products.
- The *membranes* are filled with *amniotic fluid.* The amniotic sac is also called the "bag of waters." Your baby floats inside. The fluid protects your baby and allows her to move easily. The baby also practices breathing and swallowing with the amniotic fluid.

During pregnancy, your uterus is your baby's home.

- The *uterus* (sometimes called the *womb*) is a bag of thick muscles. It's located in the pelvis behind the *bladder* (where urine collects) and in front of the *rectum.* When you're not pregnant, your uterus is about the size of a pear. During pregnancy, it expands to hold your growing baby.
- The lower part of the uterus, called the *cervix,* leads into the vagina.
- During pregnancy, a *mucous plug* in the cervix closes the opening and protects the baby.
- The *vagina* is the birth canal. During birth, the vagina stretches to allow the delivery of the baby. After birth, it returns to its previous size.

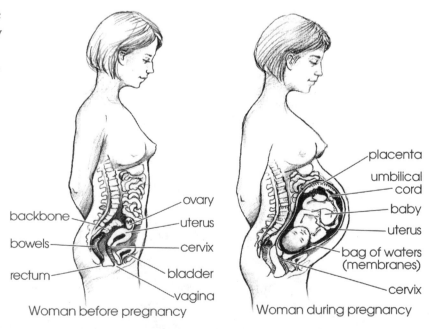

backbone · ovary
bowels · uterus
rectum · cervix
· bladder
· vagina
Woman before pregnancy

placenta
umbilical cord
baby
uterus
bag of waters (membranes)
cervix
Woman during pregnancy

> ### Jenny's Story
>
> Kyle and I started dating in high school. After graduating, he had trouble getting a good job, so he was planning to go to community college. We hadn't planned on having a baby.
>
> I was shocked when I found out I was pregnant. I thought we were being careful. Kyle was mad at first. He said he wasn't ready to be a father. But we talked about it a lot and got some good advice from family and friends about how we could manage this. They also offered to help. Now, we're starting to get excited. I know it's hard to be a parent, but I already love my baby, and he or she isn't even born yet!

When Will Your Baby Be Born?

Your *due date* is only an estimate (best guess) of when your baby will be ready to be born, but it's helpful to know. You can figure out your due date by using an online calculator or by using this formula:

Write down the first day of your last menstrual period. Then subtract 3 months from that date and add 7 days.

Date of first day of last period _____ *− 3 months* _____ *+ 7 days* _____ *= due date* _____	*For example:* *Last period started on* July 10 *− 3 months* April 10 *+ 7 days* April 17 *= due date* April 17 of the next year

An ultrasound scan can confirm how many weeks pregnant you are but can't predict exactly when your baby will come. Pregnancy lasts about 40 weeks from the first day of your last menstrual period. But some babies come early and some come late. Most babies are born within 10 days of their due dates. Expect your baby anytime from 2 weeks before to 2 weeks after your due date.

> ### Maria's Story
>
> John always wanted to be a father, and he couldn't wait for the 9 months to pass. But I felt like I needed the 9 months to get ready to be a mom. We read books and took classes together, and we talked to our friends and coworkers about what it's like to be a parent. We babysat for a friend—we called their daughter our "practice baby."

What Happens during Pregnancy?

Pregnancy is divided into 3 time periods (called *trimesters*), with each time period lasting about 3 months. Most people say that pregnancy lasts 9 months. Actually, it lasts a little longer (about 40 weeks total).

How Your Baby Is Growing

To learn more details about how your baby is developing, go to www.babycenter.com/pregnancy for their guide, "Your Pregnancy, Week by Week," or visit www.lamaze.org to sign up for their weekly e-mail newsletter "Pregnancy Week by Week." You can also download Lamaze's mobile app, "Pregnancy to Parenting."

Changes in the First 3 Months of Pregnancy

This is the "forming" period for your baby. All your baby's organ systems (such as the stomach, lungs, heart, and nerves) will form and start to work. After 14 weeks of pregnancy (12 weeks after conception), this is how your baby has changed:

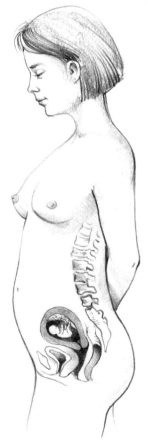

- He is about 3 inches long and weighs about 1 ounce.
- He has eyes, ears, a nose, and a mouth.
- He has arms with hands and fingers with fingerprints.
- He has legs with knees, ankles, and toes.
- He makes breathing movements but is not really breathing. (Your baby gets oxygen from you through the umbilical cord.)
- He has a heartbeat that can be heard with a special stethoscope called a Doppler.

During the first 3 months, your developing baby becomes quite active, although you probably don't feel any movements yet. His legs kick, and his arms move. He can smile and frown, suck his thumb, swallow amniotic fluid, and *urinate* (pee) into the amniotic fluid. The fluid stays clean because it's refreshed many times each day.

Cami's Story

As soon as I got pregnant, I started eating breakfast every day and drinking decaf instead of my usual coffee. I started going to bed earlier. I felt like I was changing into a parent, and my life was different than it was before. But we hadn't told our friends and coworkers yet. I was falling asleep at my desk sometimes because I was just so tired, and I was afraid my coworkers thought I was a total slacker. My friends were doing this wine tasting thing, and I had to figure out an excuse not to drink. I told them I had a big work project due.

For you, the first 3 months of pregnancy is a time when your body and mind get used to being pregnant and the effects of increased hormones. Although the physical and emotional changes may feel big to you, other people may not even notice that you're pregnant. On page 15 are some physical changes you may experience:

- no menstrual periods
- nausea and vomiting (called *morning sickness*, but may occur at any time during the day)
- feeling tired and sleepy
- frequent peeing
- more mucus (called *discharge*) from your vagina (but not bad-smelling discharge)
- changes in your breasts (which are preparing for breastfeeding): your breasts get bigger, your nipples may tingle and feel tender, and the area around each nipple (called the *areola*) gets darker
- by the end of the first 3 months, the placenta is complete, and your uterus will be about the size of a grapefruit

Finding out you're pregnant can cause various emotions. You might feel some or all of these feelings:
- happiness about having a cute little baby
- excitement about becoming a parent
- sadness about having less freedom
- fear about how you and your partner might change
- doubts about how good a parent you'll be
- worry about not having enough money

Mood swings (unexpected feelings of joy or sadness) are normal in pregnancy. However, if you feel much more anxious or depressed than usual, you might have a perinatal mood disorder. (See page 127 for more information about mood disorders. They are almost as common during pregnancy as postpartum, after the birth.)

Jenny's Story

I knew something was different even before I noticed I'd missed my period. My breasts got sore. Then it was 1 thing after another. I couldn't stand certain smells, like garlic and cigarettes. I had to have Kyle's friend go outside to smoke. I fell asleep in front of the TV and riding the bus. And I felt sick to my stomach off and on during the day. My nurse told me all those things were signs of a healthy early pregnancy and my body changing to support my baby's needs. Luckily, all of this got better after a couple of months.

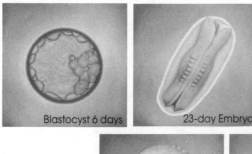

Blastocyst 6 days

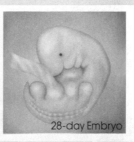

23-day Embryo

28-day Embryo

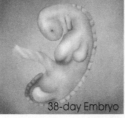

38-day Embryo

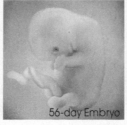

56-day Embryo

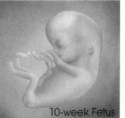

10-week Fetus

Changes in the Second 3 Months of Pregnancy

The second trimester lasts from week 15 to week 27. This is the development period for your baby, when her organs and body parts grow and mature. Your baby is still tiny and not ready to be born. By the end of the 24th week, this is how your baby has changed:

- She is 10–13 inches long and weighs about 1½ pounds.
- She has a strong heartbeat.
- She begins to have fingernails and toenails, hair, eyelashes, and eyebrows.
- She has a strong grip and is able to suck her thumb.
- She gets the hiccups. She can roll around and move her arms and legs.
- She begins to hear.

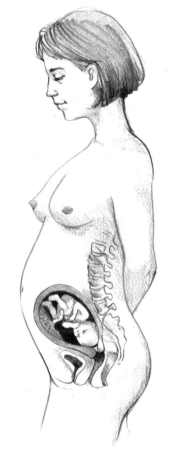

Maria's Story

After 3 or 4 months, I had more energy. I got my appetite back too. I started craving hot peppers. Sometimes peppers were all I wanted to eat! Nothing fit, so I wore John's shirts and left the top button of my jeans undone when I was at home. At work, I felt fat until I got some maternity clothes. The best part of all was near the end of second trimester, when I started feeling our baby move! At first, it was a little fluttery feeling. Pretty soon, I knew it was our baby kicking and rolling around.

You'll probably feel fine during these middle months of pregnancy. Nausea usually goes away, and you have more energy. You might notice some of these new signs of your growing pregnancy:

- food cravings
- sharp pains in your lower belly or hip when you sneeze or stand up quickly
- hard bowel movements (*constipation*)
- a dark line (*linea nigra*) on your belly (*abdomen*) up to your bellybutton
- darkening of the skin around your eyes and nose (called the *mask of pregnancy*)
- stuffy or bloody nose
- bleeding from your gums when you brush or floss
- weight gain (up to 1 pound per week)
- your baby's movements (a light tapping feeling that may remind you of gas bubbles); a first-time mom may not feel these until week 24 or so, but women who have had babies before feel them sooner

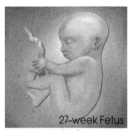

27-week Fetus

- *Braxton-Hicks contractions* (tightening of your uterus muscles) begin to be noticeable late in second trimester. You might be able to feel the contraction happening, or see that you're having a contraction if your belly changes shape as your uterus presses against it. Or you might need to put your fingers on your belly to feel if your uterus is hard. Braxton-Hicks contractions are normal in pregnancy. However, sometimes contractions like these are a sign of having your baby too early (*preterm labor*). See page 30 to learn about preterm labor.

At this time, your uterus is larger, and you now look pregnant. Some women enjoy how they look and feel, while others do not. You may experience some of these thoughts and emotions:

- think you're too fat, especially if you're having trouble moving around
- notice changes in your feelings about sex
- feel more dependent on others
- be more interested in babies and parenting
- feel creative
- daydream and dream more at night

By the end of 6 months, your pregnancy seems more real to your family and friends. Now you look bigger. You can feel the baby move, and so can others when they touch your growing belly.

Changes in the Third 3 Months of Pregnancy

This is the growth period for your baby as he prepares for life outside your uterus. His lungs mature, and you pass antibodies to him, which will help him to not get sick. By week 35, most babies turn to be head down in the uterus. By the end of 40 weeks of pregnancy, here's how your baby has changed:

- He is about 20 inches long and weighs about 7–8 pounds.
- He is fully developed.
- He kicks and wiggles but doesn't turn and roll very much.
- He has noticeable times of being awake and being asleep.
- He hears sounds and voices.

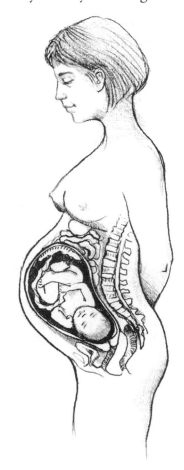

It's loud in the uterus. Your baby is used to the sounds of your heart beating, your stomach gurgling, and the blood circulating through your placenta. You may notice that sudden, loud noises make him jump. Your baby can hear your voice. You or your partner can try talking or singing to him. Sometimes he will respond by kicking or changing position.

During the last 3 months of pregnancy, your uterus grows until it reaches up to your ribs. Many of the common changes at this time come from having a big belly. The others are caused by hormones. You may notice these changes:

- Your sense of balance shifts, and you may feel clumsy.
- It's hard to breathe deeply.
- Backaches bother you.
- The veins in your legs seem bigger.
- Your ankles swell.
- You have painful swelling of blood vessels in your rectum (*hemorrhoids*).
- You pee more frequently.
- Red *stretch marks* may appear on your belly, thighs, or breasts. (They fade to shiny lines after the birth.)
- You probably have trouble sleeping.

Cami's Story

I was surprised at how big I got in the last couple of months of pregnancy. I got big red stretch marks on my belly. I'd hoped I wouldn't get them. It was August, and I was hot all the time. I went swimming and waded in the lake a lot. At night, I'd keep the fan pointed at me. I loved feeling the baby move. I called him Thumper. I couldn't wait till my due date. I wanted to meet our baby and stop feeling so fat and hot! But at the same time, I was anxious about birth. I still had a hard time imagining this big baby coming out of me!

Toward the end of pregnancy, your uterus tightens (*contracts*) more. These *prelabor contractions* help increase blood flow in your uterus. They also press your baby downward onto your cervix, making it softer and thinner. (See page 64 for more about how labor starts.)

About 2 weeks before the birth, your baby may drop lower in your pelvis. This is called *engagement* or *lightening*. You may find it easier to breathe and have less heartburn after your baby drops. However, you may need to go to the bathroom more as your baby's head presses on your bladder.

Expectant parents often have mixed feelings during this time in pregnancy. You may have some of these thoughts and reactions or all of them:

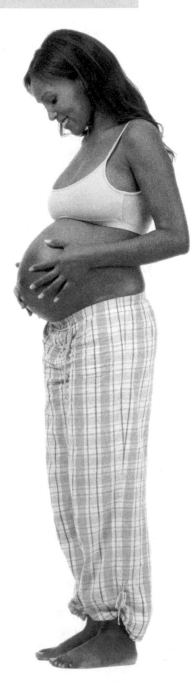

- be ready for pregnancy to be over
- need more help from others
- have concerns about becoming a parent
- think more about your own parents and how they cared for you
- be excited about having a new baby

All these feelings are normal. Talking about your concerns with someone who's a good listener (your partner, a relative, your caregiver, or a friend) can help you feel better.

Near the end of pregnancy, you may think and worry more about labor, birth, and the baby. By taking childbirth classes, you and your partner can learn more about birth, baby care, and breastfeeding. You worry less when you're prepared for these experiences.

Note to Fathers and Partners

Waiting for your baby to be born can be exciting but difficult. It sometimes takes a while to get used to the idea of being a parent, especially if the pregnancy was a surprise.

A parent-to-be thinks about all the changes that will come. Here are some things you may worry about:

- **Losing your freedom.** You know that babies need constant care, and you'll need to help more around your home.
- **Having enough money.** You may feel as though you're more responsible for supporting your family.
- **The possible death of your partner or baby.** This may lead you to be very protective of your partner. You may also worry about your own death.
- **Feeling unwanted.** You may feel that your pregnant partner doesn't love you as much since before the pregnancy. At the same time, you're expected to do more for your partner. It helps to talk to each other about these feelings. Your partner may not know how you're feeling.
- **Your role during labor and birth.** You may wonder, "What will I do during labor? Will I faint?" Taking childbirth classes, reading books, and talking with other fathers or partners will help prepare you for your role during labor and birth. Also, having another person at the birth may take the pressure off you. (For more information about labor support, see pages 68 and 87–88.)
- **Physical changes and discomforts.** Some partners gain weight or have food cravings, nausea, or backaches—just like their pregnant partners. It's how you may show sympathy for your partner.
- **Your own childhood.** As you think about your baby, you'll remember your childhood—both the good and the tough times. You may remember some things that happened to you that you don't want your child to go through. You may also look forward to reliving some of the fun parts of being a kid.
- **Newborn care.** During pregnancy, take newborn care classes with your partner, babysit for friends, watch families at the park or mall, and ask advice from other parents. Learning about children and parenting helps you be a good parent from day 1.

John's Story

At the beginning, it was almost hard to remember that Maria was pregnant—she didn't seem any different from before, even though she kept telling me she felt different. But when her belly got bigger, it started feeling more real. I went to her 20 week ultrasound with her, and it was so cool to see our baby girl for the first time! We started buying stuff to get ready for the baby and talking more to our friends about their kids. Once I could feel the baby kick, I started singing to Maria's belly at night. I feel goofy doing it, but I know the baby can hear me, and I want her to get to know me. I'm a little freaked out about the birth and how I'll help Maria get through it, but I know I can handle being a dad.

What about Sex during Pregnancy?

Your feelings about sex may change during pregnancy. These feelings are normal and common:

- Some people feel beautiful and sexual during pregnancy, while others feel clumsy and fat.
- One person may feel loved by a caring partner, while another may be alone or in a difficult relationship.
- One person's partner may feel turned off by her growing belly, while another may love it.
- Body changes, such as nausea, tiredness, or breast tenderness, will affect your desire for sex. Some people don't want to have sex at all when they're pregnant; others do.
- Some partners worry about harming you or the baby during sex.

Talk about your sex life with your partner. Try to understand and respect each other's feelings. What you find exciting may change. Some people don't want to have sex but want to be hugged, cuddled, and loved. If you want to have sex, it's okay to have sex. You may find you have uterine contractions (cramps) when you have an orgasm. These are normal, and they don't cause problems for the baby during a healthy pregnancy.

Sex may be more comfortable if you don't lie on your back with your partner's weight on your belly. Try other positions, such as lying on your sides with him or her behind you, or your partner on his or her back with you on top.

If you have a new partner during pregnancy or your partner does, remember to use safer sex methods, such as condoms and dental dams. Your partner might have a disease (such as genital herpes, HIV, or genital warts) that could spread to you during sex and affect your baby.

Your caregiver may say that you should *not* have sexual intercourse if any of the following is true:

- You're at risk for preterm labor (labor occurring more than 3 weeks before your due date).
- You've had vaginal bleeding during pregnancy.
- You have painful cramps after intercourse. (Mild cramps are normal.)

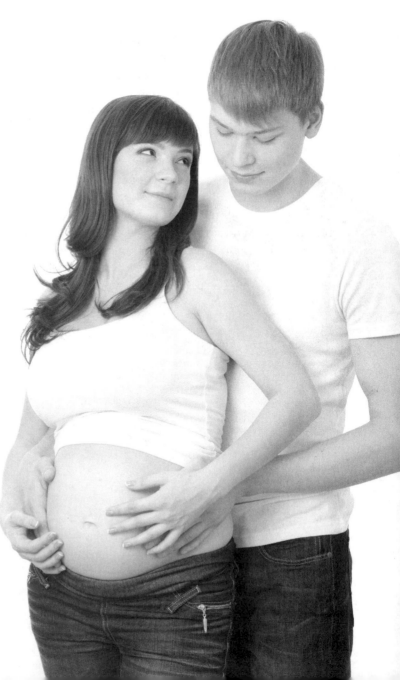

Special Concerns You May Have

Some people have special questions about how their age, relationships, history, and current situations may affect their pregnancy. Here are questions they may ask.

Does Your Age Make a Difference?

If you're a teenager, your chances of a healthy pregnancy and birth are good. Because your body is still growing, it's especially important for you to eat well for you and your baby and to stay away from drugs, alcohol, and tobacco. You'll need extra support with school and life planning. Ask for help from understanding friends and family, a school counselor, or a public health nurse.

If you're over 35, you have a higher risk of high blood pressure, gestational diabetes, preterm labor, and birth defects. You may have more testing than a younger parent would.

How healthy you are is more important than how old you are. Beginning pregnancy in the best possible health, taking good care of yourself in pregnancy, and getting good prenatal care helps you and your baby.

What If You Already Have Another Child?

When you're pregnant again, it may not seem as exciting as your first pregnancy. It may be harder to find time to rest. Also, going to doctor or midwife appointments may be more difficult when you have to take a child with you. Pregnancy changes take place more easily in a body that's done it before.

- You feel the baby's movements earlier.
- Your uterus may get bigger sooner.
- You may notice more prelabor contractions toward the end of pregnancy.

You may worry, "Will it be harder than last time?" and "Will I be able to handle labor pain?" If a past birth experience was scary or if you had problems, you may be especially worried. This is normal. Talking about it with your partner and caregivers may help. If your caregivers know about your worries, they may be able to think of ways to help you feel better. You can also take a refresher birth class.

In general, second labors are faster and less painful than first labors. Pushing may hurt a little more, just because it happens more quickly.

Many second-time parents wonder if they have enough love for another child. Or you may worry that you'll love your first child less after the new baby arrives. These are common worries. Remember that you can love many people. You don't run out of love. You can love another baby without taking love away from your older child.

You may also wonder how your older child will react to the new baby. (See page 172 for more on this issue.)

Tanya's Story

I didn't enjoy pregnancy as much this time. Lifting my daughter and bending over to pick up toys made my back hurt. Jason and I didn't talk much about my pregnancy. We spent more time thinking about what it would be like to have 2 children. We also wondered how Molly would like having a brother or sister.

What If You're Expecting Twins, Triplets, or More?

When a woman is carrying more than 1 baby, it's called a *multiple pregnancy*. A sign of multiple pregnancy is hearing 2 or more heartbeats. An ultrasound scanner (a machine that uses sound waves to see inside you) proves that you're really having more than 1 baby.

Expecting multiples is exciting and stressful. Most people think twins and triplets are special, even though they're a lot more work. Growing more than 1 baby puts extra demands on your body. You gain weight more quickly, and your uterus grows faster. Here's what you may need to do differently than someone pregnant with 1 baby:

- Eat more food.
- Get more rest.
- Go to an *obstetrician* (a doctor with special training in treating childbirth problems) instead of a midwife or family doctor.
- Prepare for the possibility of a preterm birth.

If you're expecting more than 1 baby, you may want to talk to other parents of multiples. (For more information, see Help for You and Your Baby on page 180.)

What If Your Partner Is Not the Biological Father?

If you conceived the pregnancy with a donor egg or sperm, you or your partner may have a hard time coming to terms with the fact that your baby is not your biological child.

If you're in a new relationship since becoming pregnant or if your partner is not the biological parent, that can be stressful for both of you. Your partner may feel like the pregnancy is "yours," not "ours." Or your partner may not be sure what his or her role is in supporting you and caring for the baby. This is especially true if the biological parent is still involved.

Talk with your partner about these feelings. Discuss what you would each like to have happen and come to an agreement.

What If You're Lesbian or Transgender?

If you have a female partner or if you or your partner are transgender, you deserve a supportive caregiver. Visit http://glma.org to find a caregiver or ask for referrals from a local LGBTQ organization. Connect with other queer parents, either local or online, for support. Write a detailed birth plan that includes what pronouns you prefer and what you would like to be called (mama and mommy, pregnant dad, and so on). Ask your caregiver for support with hospital staff, such as sharing your birth plan in advance.

What's It Like Being a Single Parent?

Pregnancy and parenthood may be difficult when you don't have a partner. Being a parent is hard work, and it's a job usually shared by 2 people. There may be times when you wonder if you can do it. You may feel lonely and wish you had a dependable partner. At other times, you may be thankful that you don't have to deal with a demanding or unkind partner.

It's especially difficult if you don't have family and friends to help you. This is a time to reach out to others for help, emotional support, and, possibly, financial support. Search online for single parent support groups in your area.

Is Pregnancy Different If You Have Been Abused?

When someone has been physically, sexually, or emotionally abused, even long ago, it can cause unexpected reactions during pregnancy, birth, and *postpartum* (after the birth). Being hurt or abused by a more powerful person may make it hard to trust another powerful person. For example, you may not trust your doctor or midwife. A victim of sexual abuse may find vaginal exams or nakedness extremely upsetting. Some people who have been abused believe that the experience of having a vaginal birth would be unbearable.

Talk with your caregivers about your feelings. This may help you receive health care that's more sensitive to your needs. Consider talking to a counselor about your experiences. A helpful resource is the book *When Survivors Give Birth* by Penny Simkin.

What If You're Being Abused Now?

No one deserves to be beaten, yelled at, or forced to have sex. No one deserves to feel powerless or trapped by a partner. If this is happening to you, you must protect yourself and your baby. Though you may feel like you can't get out of your situation, at least try to find places or people who can help you. Memorize the phone number for the National Domestic Violence Hotline 800-799-SAFE and call if you need help.

What If You Plan to Have Your Baby Adopted by Another Family?

The decision to give your baby to an adoptive family is one that many women think about, especially if they're not ready or able to raise a child. It's not an easy decision. It helps to talk it over with someone who isn't trying to make you decide either way. This person can help you think about what's best for both the baby and you. Whatever you decide, you'll need support.

When you're planning on adoption, you'll experience the feelings and changes of pregnancy, but the joy may not be there. The weeks after the birth can also be difficult. Rely on your support system to help you cope with this challenging time.

You may want to write a letter to the baby about the pregnancy and birth. Along with a baby toy or present, this could be a special gift from you. Or you may choose an open adoption, which could allow you to have ongoing contact with the baby.

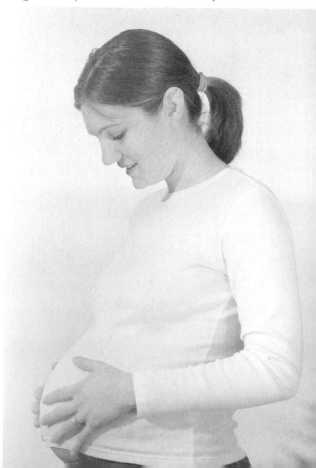

CHAPTER 3

Health Care during Pregnancy

Early in pregnancy (or before you are pregnant), you will choose a health caregiver for pregnancy and birth, and choose where you want to have the baby. During pregnancy, plan on regular visits and recommended tests to check on the health of you and your baby. If any problems come up, early treatment will help you and your baby remain as healthy as possible.

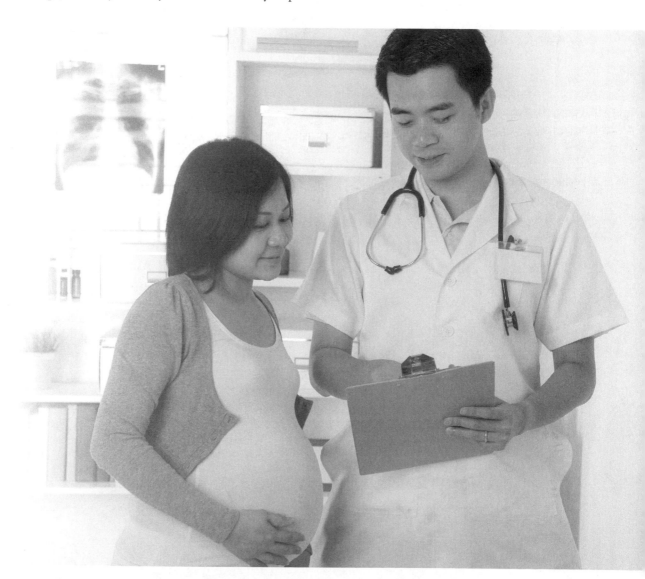

Prenatal Care

Prenatal care is the health care you get while you're pregnant. A doctor, midwife, or nurse provides prenatal care. You'll have many appointments and some tests during your pregnancy. Here's what these help your caregiver to do:

- check on your health
- check on how well your baby is growing
- find any problems and treat them before they become serious
- offer advice on how to care for yourself and your growing baby

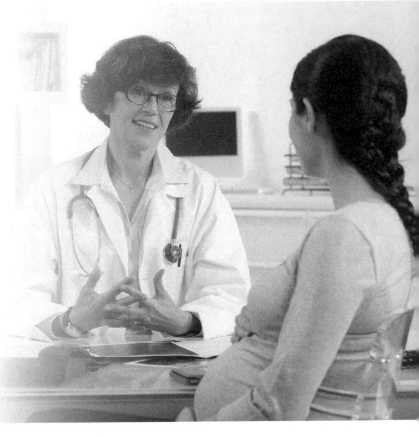

At your first prenatal visit, you'll have a complete physical examination and several laboratory tests. You'll be asked about past illnesses and surgeries. Make sure your caregiver knows about any medications you're taking. To get the most from your visits, make a list before you go of the questions and concerns you'd like to discuss with your caregiver.

During most of your pregnancy, you'll have appointments once a month. As you get closer to your due date, they'll be scheduled every 2 weeks or every week. Try not to miss your checkups. If you have trouble getting time off work, finding child care, or getting to the clinic, you may think about skipping one. Instead, try to find someone to take you. You can ask a public health nurse about getting help with transportation or child care. If you do miss an appointment, call the clinic and schedule another time.

If you have to take older children, time spent in the waiting room may seem to last forever. Bring toys for the children and a snack for all of you. Ask your partner or a friend to go with you.

Tanya's Story

For Molly's birth, I went to an Ob-Gyn that a friend recommended, who delivered at the hospital closest to my house. It was fine. But sometimes when I had prenatal checkups, I had to wait in the waiting room for a long time, and appointments were pretty short, since he had a lot of patients. But he was nice, and I got good care. This time, I'm seeing a midwife. She schedules appointments that are a lot longer, and she sits and talks with me at each one about how things are going and what my hopes are for the birth. It's nice to have a chance to ask all my questions.

What Are Your Choices for a Caregiver?

If you have health insurance, you need to find out what caregivers are available to you. If you have Medicaid, find out who accepts Medicaid for maternity care. If you don't have insurance and can't afford to pay, check with your public health department or a social worker at a nearby hospital about help with prenatal care costs. Learn more about health-care coverage at http://healthcare.gov.

Then ask friends, family, and coworkers for their advice on which caregiver to choose. On page 177, we list resources for finding caregivers. Although all caregivers can help you have a safe birth, there are important differences between them. Choosing the right caregiver and birthplace for you can help you have the satisfying birth you are hoping for. Learn more in the *Great Starts Guide*, found at http://www.parenttrust.org/web-store/books.

Options for Caregivers for Pregnancy and Birth
• Obstetricians are medical doctors who care for expectant parents during pregnancy and birth and for several weeks afterward. They are the best option for high-risk pregnancies.
• Family doctors provide medical care for the whole family, including new babies. Some care for expectant parents during pregnancy and birth.
• Midwives provide very safe and supportive care for expectant parents who have a low risk of problems during pregnancy or birth. Most are certified nurse-midwives (CNMs) or state-licensed midwives (LMs).
• Nurse practitioners provide care in a clinic along with doctors or midwives. They see expectant parents before and after birth. They don't provide care during childbirth.
• Naturopaths are natural medicine doctors, not medical doctors. Some are also midwives and care for clients during pregnancy, childbirth, and postpartum.

Where Will Your Baby Be Born?

Most babies in the United States and Canada are born in hospitals. You may or may not be able to choose your hospital. It depends on your health-care coverage and where you live. To learn more about a specific hospital, take a hospital tour (see page 56). Also, talk to friends about the different hospitals in your area.

Some women want to give birth at home, where they feel most comfortable. Others choose an out-of-hospital birth center, which offers a homelike setting. Caregivers in both settings have equipment with them to handle the most common emergencies. If there are problems in labor, such as a very long labor that's not progressing or you want pain medicine, you would transfer to a hospital.

You may choose to have an out-of-hospital birth only if you have a *low-risk pregnancy* (one with no major problems) and expect a normal labor and birth. Women who have a planned out-of-hospital birth with a trained caregiver typically are very satisfied with their birth experience. The cost of an out-of-hospital birth is usually much lower than the cost of hospital care. Check your health insurance or your local health department to see if the costs are covered.

Cami's Story

Because of my age, I knew I had a higher chance of problems than a younger mom. So I planned to choose an OB and a hospital so I'd have all the help I needed if any issues came up. But I wanted the birth to be as natural as possible. So I talked to friends who had babies, and I read online reviews, and I searched online to find out about the different hospitals in town. Then Chris and I toured two hospitals to find the best match for the birth I was hoping for.

What Prenatal Tests Are Usually Done?

During pregnancy, you'll have tests to find out how you and your baby are doing.

These tests are common during pregnancy:

- urine tests and blood tests (used first to be sure that you are pregnant, used later to check for diabetes and to see if all your organs are working well)
- blood pressure checks
- weight checks
- pelvic exams (your caregiver checks for changes in your cervix by placing 2 fingers in your vagina)
- abdominal exams (your caregiver feels your belly to check on your baby's growth and position)
- listening to your baby's heartbeat (*fetal heart rate or FHR*)

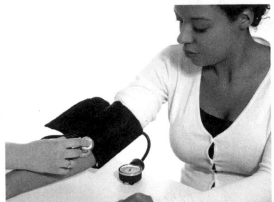

If one of those tests shows a possible problem, then your caregiver may order some of these more specific tests:

- *ultrasound scan* (sound waves are used to create a video image of the uterus and baby)
- *integrated prenatal screening* is a combination of an ultrasound and blood tests to see if your baby has common birth defects
- *amniocentesis* (fluid from the uterus is withdrawn and tested)
- vaginal fluid collection and testing
- *non-stress test* (your caregiver listens to how the baby's heart rate responds when the baby moves within the uterus)
- genetic testing (see page 6)

To learn more about all these tests, go to http://www.marchofdimes.com and look in the pregnancy section. Whenever a test is recommended, you can ask these questions to help you decide whether to have the test:

- What is the test? How is it done?
- Benefits: What will you learn by having the test? How will the results change your care or the decisions you need to make?
- Risks: Could the test harm you or your baby?
- Options: Are there other tests you could have instead?

When you are given the results of a test, ask these questions:

- Are we certain there is a problem? (A *diagnostic test* can tell for certain that you or baby definitely has the condition you were tested for. A *screening test* just says whether it's likely that you or baby have the condition. Some tests are very accurate, but some can give false results.)
- What next: Do we need to do more testing now, or are there treatments that are recommended based on the results of this test?

Note to Fathers and Partners

Plan to go to prenatal care appointments with your partner as often as you can. This shows that you care about your partner and the pregnancy. Before the appointment, help come up with a list of questions for you and your partner to ask. At the appointment, make sure you pay attention and remember the answers. You will also learn about the warning signs in pregnancy and can help watch out for them.

Going to the prenatal appointments may help you feel more involved in the pregnancy. Hearing the baby's heartbeat or seeing the baby in an ultrasound may help you feel more connected to the baby as he grows.

When Should You Call Your Doctor or Midwife?

It's important to pay attention to how you feel during pregnancy. If you're worried or feel sick, call your caregiver. Also, if you have any of these warning signs, call right away. Most problems can be treated before they become serious.

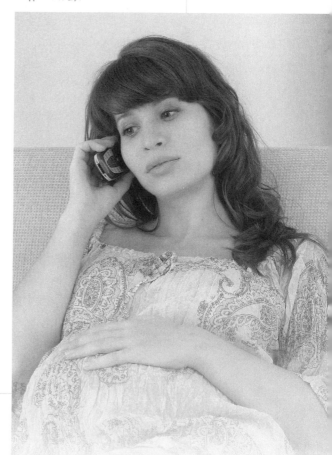

Warning Signs of Pregnancy Problems

If you notice any of the following, call your doctor or midwife right away:

- bleeding from your vagina
- leaking or a gush of water from your vagina
- tightening (contractions) or cramping in your belly that comes and goes (6 contractions per hour) or other signs of preterm labor (see page 30)
- a hard belly with constant pain (with or without vaginal bleeding)
- one or all of these signs of high blood pressure:
  - sudden swelling in your hands, feet, and face
  - severe headache that lasts for hours
  - eyesight problems (spots, flashes, blurring)
  - severe dizziness, lightheadedness, or feeling faint
- any of these signs of infection (see page 31)
- fever (a temperature of 100.4°F or 38°C or higher taken with a thermometer in your mouth)
- pain or burning while peeing
- soreness, itching, or bad smell in your vagina
- nausea and vomiting that continues even after trying all the tips on page 47
- painful, red area on your leg (or pain in your leg when standing or walking)
- no movement by your baby for 12–24 hours

Possible Pregnancy Problems

These are some of the problems that might cause the warning signs listed in the box on page 29.

Preterm Labor

If you have contractions before the 37th week of pregnancy, you may be in *preterm labor*. Babies who are born too early have more health problems than babies born on time. For this reason, it's important to prevent or stop preterm labor contractions.

How Do You Know If You're Having Preterm Labor?

Signs of preterm labor are very similar to normal sensations in pregnancy. Watch for these symptoms:
* uterine contractions that are frequent and regular (see page 65 to learn what contractions feel like)
* cramps in your lower belly
* low, dull backache that makes it hard to sit still or get comfortable
* pressure in your lower belly or thighs (pelvic heaviness)
* more bowel movements (BMs) than usual or diarrhea
* sudden increase or change in vaginal discharge (more mucus, water, or mucus with blood)
* general feeling that something isn't right

Call your doctor or midwife if you're having contractions every 10 minutes or less (this means 6 or more contractions in an hour for one hour or longer), and you've had other symptoms of preterm labor.

How Can You Stop Preterm Contractions?

If you have an infection or other problem that is causing preterm labor, your caregiver may give you medicine to treat it. If not, your caregiver may ask you to do these things to try to stop contractions:
* Drink plenty of water. Sometimes dehydration (not drinking enough water) causes contractions.
* Stay in bed or spend less time on your feet.
* Check for contractions and watch for other symptoms of labor.
* Don't have sex.
* Don't stroke or rub your nipples.

If these steps do not stop contractions, your caregiver may check to see if the contractions are changing your cervix. If so, and you are past 34 weeks, labor may be allowed to continue. If you are before 34 weeks, your baby's lungs are not yet mature. They will give you medicine to slow your labor for a few days while they also give you steroid medications to help get your baby ready to be born.

Maria's Story

When I was 6 months pregnant, I had a day where I suddenly had to pee really often—like every hour. And it burned when I peed. I guess I knew it might be an infection, but I didn't do anything about it. Then I started having a bunch of contractions. I had to go to the hospital because I was afraid the baby was coming early. It turns out I did have a bladder infection that needed to be treated. I was having contractions, but luckily they hadn't changed my cervix yet. I'm glad I went in when I did.

Infections

Certain infections during pregnancy may cause problems for you or your baby. Whether it's serious depends on when you get the infection and what it is. Some infections harm the baby only if you have them in the first 3 months (for example, rubella or German measles). Others are dangerous if you have the infection when the baby is born (for example, genital herpes). In addition, some can cause problems at any time during pregnancy (for example, HIV). However, just because you get an infection doesn't mean your baby has been infected or harmed.

Make sure to tell your caregiver if you have any of these signs of an infection:

- fever
- sores around your vagina
- unusual vaginal discharge
- pain when peeing
- rash
- vomiting
- feeling sick

When you see your caregiver, you can be tested and treated, if necessary. Treatment for an infection depends on the type of germ (bacteria or virus) that's causing it. If bacteria are causing your infection, you'll probably get an *antibiotic* (a germ-fighting drug).

Diabetes

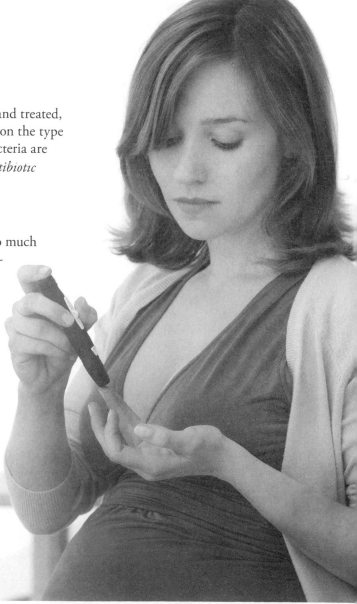

Diabetes means that you have a problem with too much sugar in your blood. It's because you have a problem making *insulin*, a hormone that helps your body use *glucose* (sugar) for energy. *Gestational diabetes* starts during pregnancy. About the 26th week of pregnancy, you'll have a glucose test to check for diabetes. For the test, you'll drink a really sweet beverage and then have your blood taken. Eat a healthy diet and get plenty of rest in the days before your glucose test for best results.

Whether you have diabetes before pregnancy or get it during pregnancy, you'll need to take special care to control your blood sugar levels. This will help prevent problems for your baby, such as being too big, having low blood sugar, or developing birth defects. Treatment includes a special diet, regular exercise, and in some cases pills or insulin shots. Learn more at http://www.niddk.nih.gov/health-information/health-topics/Diabetes/gestational-diabetes.

High Blood Pressure

In pregnancy, *high blood pressure* (hypertension) can cause serious problems for you and your baby. *Gestational hypertension* is a type of high blood pressure that starts in pregnancy. Some women also have *preeclampsia,* which is high blood pressure plus problems with organs, like the kidney or liver. Hypertension makes it so that not enough blood gets to the uterus, which means less oxygen and nourishment for the baby.

Because it's important to detect this issue, your blood pressure is taken at every prenatal visit. Finding out that you have high blood pressure early allows your caregiver to treat it so it doesn't become dangerous. If not treated, it could worsen and cause seizures, coma, or even death of the mother. Once your baby is born, your blood pressure will likely return to normal.

What Are the Symptoms of Gestational Hypertension?

You might have some of the following signs. If you notice any of them, call your caregiver as soon as possible:

- sudden swelling (*edema*) or puffiness, especially in your hands and face
- rapid weight gain
- nausea or vomiting in the second half of pregnancy
- headaches that won't stop, blurred vision, spots before your eyes
- pain in your upper belly near your stomach, shoulder, or lower back

At your prenatal visits, your caregivers check for these other signs:

- blood pressure over 140/90 (mild hypertension) or above 160/110 (severe hypertension)
- protein in your urine

How Can You Control High Blood Pressure?

If you have hypertension, treatment depends on how serious it is. You may simply need to lie down and rest more. Reducing stress in your life may be helpful. Also, try the relaxation techniques on pages 81–83. Your caregiver may ask you to take your blood pressure at home and count baby's movements once every day.

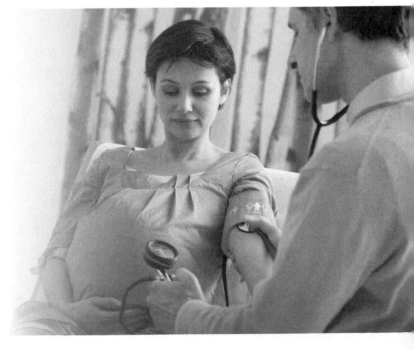

You may get medicine to help lower your blood pressure or prevent harmful effects. It's important that you follow your caregiver's advice. Both you and your baby will be healthier. Your caregiver may recommend starting your labor at 37 weeks. If you have severe preeclampsia, you may be put in the hospital for medication and may have the baby even earlier.

Problems with the Placenta

In *placenta previa*, the placenta lies over the cervix.
An ultrasound scan alerts your caregiver of this rare
condition. Often, a placenta that covers the cervix
in early pregnancy moves and causes no problems
later. But if the placenta stays over the cervix, a
cesarean birth will be done before labor begins.
(See pages 109–111 for more on cesarean.) Sometimes placenta previa causes vaginal bleeding in
the last month of pregnancy.

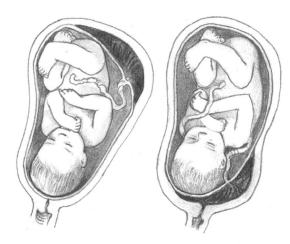

Normal Placement   Placenta Previa

With a *placental abruption*, the placenta begins
to pull away from the uterus in the last months of
pregnancy or during labor. This is rare. The symptoms
are vaginal bleeding, a hard uterus, and severe abdom-
inal pain. Your caregiver can tell the amount of separation by looking at an ultrasound scan.
Treatment may be bed rest if the separation is small. If the baby is in danger, a cesarean birth is done.

Conclusion

After reading this section, it may seem like every pregnant person has problems. In fact, most people
have healthy pregnancies and healthy babies. If you do have a health problem, knowing the warning
signs to watch out for will help you get early treatment.

CHAPTER 4
Staying Healthy during Pregnancy

This chapter helps you learn how to be healthy, safe, and comfortable during pregnancy. What you do (and don't do) also helps your baby to grow and develop well. You don't have to do everything perfectly all the time, but the more healthy choices you make each day, the healthier you and your baby will be. Creating a healthier lifestyle now can help you continue to make healthy choices after your baby is born.

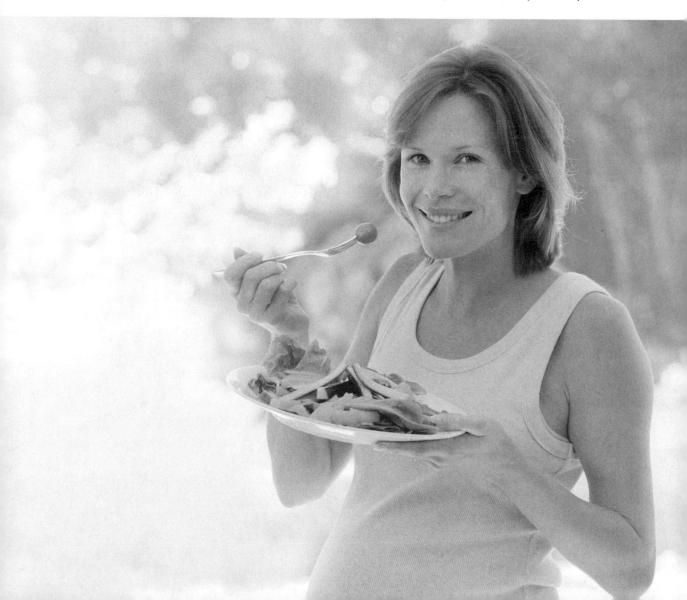

Tips for Having a Healthy Baby
• Have regular prenatal care appointments.
• Eat healthy foods and drink plenty of water.
• Exercise regularly and take care of your body.
• Get enough sleep and reduce stress.
• Don't smoke, drink alcohol, or take street drugs and try to stay away from toxic chemicals and harmful situations.
• Follow your caregiver's advice about taking medicines, and try the home remedies and simple tips we offer for handling the discomforts of pregnancy.

Note to Fathers and Partners

Even though you're not growing a baby, this pregnancy also offers you a chance to start making some healthy lifestyle changes. The healthier the habits you develop, the better your health will be while this child grows up, and the better example you'll set for him. Consider all of these options: eating better foods, exercising more, reducing stress, quitting smoking and drug use, and limiting alcohol to an occasional drink. Making these changes will help your partner feel supported and make it easier for both of you to make the same healthy choices.

Eat Well during Pregnancy

Eating good foods is important for staying healthy and growing a healthy baby. During pregnancy, your unborn baby gets nutrients from the foods you've eaten. Also, your body stores nutrients in preparation for breastfeeding.

What Are Nutrients?

Nutrients include proteins, carbohydrates, fats, vitamins, minerals, and water. They come from food, pills, and food supplements, but eating healthy whole foods is the best way to get them.

What Should You Eat?

Eating healthy foods that you cook yourself is best, even better if you can choose organic ingredients. If you are eating prepared foods that others have made, try to choose the ones that are less processed—more like food you could make yourself, and less like something designed by a scientist. Choose foods with less added salt, fat, and sugar, and more whole grains, fruits, and vegetables.

    Be sure to eat a variety of foods:

- Vegetables (3–3½ cups): Eat many different types of veggies. Greens, orange veggies (such as squash and sweet potatoes), dried peas and beans, beets, and mushrooms are all good choices. Generally, the

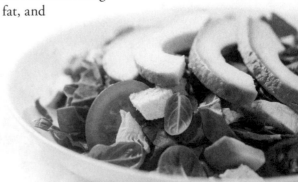

stronger the color, the more nutrients. Dark green veggies, such as broccoli, kale, and spinach, are healthier than light green lettuce.

- Fruits (2–2½ cups): Eat a variety. With fruits and vegetables, fresh is the healthiest choice, frozen is the next best, followed by dried and then canned. Very processed foods, such as fruit snacks and chips or crackers with vegetables added, have fewer nutrients.
- Grains (8–10 ounces): The best choices are brown rice, oatmeal, quinoa, and other whole grains. Eat less white rice and foods made with white flour, such as bread, flour tortillas, noodles, crackers, and cereal.
- Dairy products that provide calcium (3 servings): Choices include milk, cheese, yogurt, and foods that contain milk. You need more calcium when pregnant. If you're not able to eat milk products, get calcium from canned fish with bones, tofu, dried beans (white beans and black-eyed peas), chia seeds, greens (collard, kale, bok choy, seaweed), almonds, and calcium-fortified products or calcium supplements.

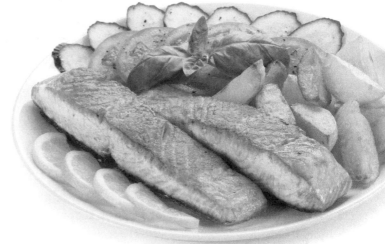

- Protein foods (6–7 ounces): Examples include meat, poultry, fish, nuts, eggs, or beans. You need more protein when pregnant. For meat and poultry, choose low-fat options or trim extra fat and cook well. If you are vegetarian, be careful to get the calcium and protein you need. If you're vegan, you will need to take a B_{12} supplement.
- Liquids: Try to drink 8 glasses (64 ounces) of water a day along with milk or juice. You know you're drinking enough if your pee is very pale yellow.
- Healthy fats: Good choices include olive oil, canola oil, avocado, nuts, fatty fish, or flaxseed. Eating the recommended amount of healthy fat is good for you and your baby.
- Take a daily prenatal vitamin with folic acid and iron.
- Try to stay away from foods that aren't healthy, such as chips, cake, cookies, candy, and soft drinks.

Examples of Serving Sizes	
Vegetables	1 cup (2 cups of leafy greens count as 1 cup of vegetables)
Fruits	1 whole fruit, 1 cup of cut-up fruit, or ½ cup of dried fruit
Grains	1 slice of bread, ½ bagel, 1 cup of cereal, or ½ cup of rice or pasta
Dairy products	1 cup of milk or yogurt, or 1½-inch cube of cheese
Protein foods	1 ounce of meat, poultry, or fish; 1 egg; or ¼ cup of nuts or cooked beans

(*Note*: These amounts are right for a pregnant woman who is 5 feet 4 inches tall and 160 pounds before pregnancy. To get the right amount for you, and to learn more about healthy eating, go to www.myplate.gov.)

At the beginning of pregnancy, you don't need to eat more food than you normally would (unless you're pregnant with twins or triplets). Add just 200 extra calories in your second trimester and 400 calories in your third trimester. (This isn't a lot of extra food. Examples of 100 calories include 1 glass of milk or 1 tablespoon of peanut butter or 1 apple.)

If you need help with getting healthy food, contact your state agency of the Women, Infants, and Children (WIC) program. You can find your state's toll-free number by visiting www.fns.usda.gov/wic. If you're pregnant and your income is below a certain level, WIC supplies some healthy food.

What Should You Be Careful about Eating or Drinking?

Caffeine

Coffee, tea, colas, and some other soft drinks contain caffeine. Some over-the-counter drugs for headaches and colds have caffeine too. Check the labels. Also, chocolate has a chemical that's similar to caffeine.

There are problems with taking too much caffeine in pregnancy. Caffeine can change your baby's heart rate, just as it may affect yours. It reduces calcium and water, and increases stress hormones, which cause blood vessels to get smaller. This may decrease oxygen and nutrients for your baby. Limit the number of caffeine drinks to 1–2 cups (8–16 ounces) a day during pregnancy.

Herbs and Supplements

Many herbal products and food *supplements* (anything added to your regular diet, including vitamins and minerals) are now available in drugstores. Some are helpful, but others may be harmful. The word *natural* does not always mean "safe." Talk to your caregiver first before taking anything.

Nonfood Substances

Food cravings are common in pregnancy and aren't harmful. Many women crave pickles, ice cream, and spicy foods. However, some women want to eat nonfood items that might not be safe: things such as dirt, ashes, charcoal, and mothballs. Eating these things isn't good for you or your baby. If you have an urge to eat nonfood (called *pica*) or to sniff harmful chemical fumes, talk to your caregiver.

Harmful Germs and Chemicals in Foods

During pregnancy, you shouldn't eat foods that might carry germs that are dangerous for your baby. For example, you should avoid eating raw fish and shellfish and undercooked meats or luncheon meats. Avoid soft cheeses that aren't *pasteurized* (check the label).

Some fish, such as shark and swordfish, shouldn't be eaten in pregnancy. They contain large amounts of mercury, which is dangerous to unborn babies and children. Other fish, such as tuna and halibut, have smaller amounts of mercury and can be eaten about once a week. Salmon, tilapia, sole, pollock, and trout are low in mercury. They can be eaten about twice a week. To learn more about these possible hazards and others, check out the fact sheets at http://www.mothertobaby.org.

How Much Weight Should You Gain during Pregnancy?

Gaining a healthy amount of weight will increase your likelihood of having a healthy baby. If you begin pregnancy underweight, you'll want to gain 28–40 pounds. If you begin at a normal weight, gain 20–35 pounds. Weight gain is usually slow in early pregnancy, just 2–4 pounds in the first 3 months. Later in pregnancy, you'll gain about 1 pound a week.

If you begin pregnancy overweight, you may need to gain only 15–25 pounds. If you are obese, less than 15 pounds is ideal. You may not need to gain weight till midpregnancy, and after that, gain just ½ pound a week. Gaining less than that may be okay if your baby is healthy and will help reduce the complications you have due to weight.

Many women have back pain in late pregnancy from the weight of the baby. To prevent this, try to have good posture (stand up straight) and do pelvic tilt exercises (see page 48).

Stand tall with your...

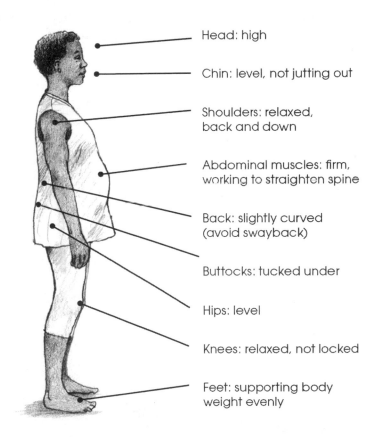

Head: high

Chin: level, not jutting out

Shoulders: relaxed, back and down

Abdominal muscles: firm, working to straighten spine

Back: slightly curved (avoid swayback)

Buttocks: tucked under

Hips: level

Knees: relaxed, not locked

Feet: supporting body weight evenly

Exercise to Stay Healthy

Exercise strengthens your muscles to support your pregnancy. Exercise helps with discomforts like back pain and swollen ankles. Exercise also reduces stress and increases your energy and sense of well-being.

What kind of exercise should you do? *Low-impact exercise* is easiest on your joints. This means no jumping or bouncing. Good exercises include walking quickly, bike riding, swimming, water exercise, and other low-impact exercises. Many women enjoy yoga or tai chi during pregnancy. These practices help with strength, flexibility, balance, and relaxation.

Aerobic Exercise

Aerobic exercise speeds up your heart rate and makes you breathe faster. Start slowly and gently. Here's what a good aerobic exercise program for a pregnant person looks like:

1. At least 5 minutes of warm-up (slow, smooth movements and stretching)
2. About 15–30 minutes of moderate to vigorous aerobic exercise
3. At least 5 minutes of cool-down (mild activity while your heart rate returns to normal)

How to Exercise Safely
These tips will help you avoid injury and get the most benefit:
• Exercise every day, if possible, for at least 30 minutes.
• Drink plenty of water and eat enough calories.
• Avoid strain and exhaustion. Can you pass the talk test? (If you're gasping and can't talk, you're exercising too hard. Slow down until you can talk comfortably.)
• Stop if you feel pain or have a headache, nausea, trouble breathing, dizziness, vaginal bleeding, or strong uterine contractions.
• Avoid getting overheated. Don't exercise in hot, humid weather or when you have a fever.

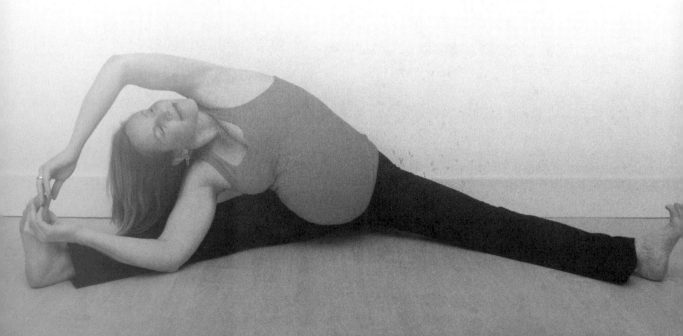

Sports

Pregnancy is not a good time to start a new sport that requires good balance. If you're already playing a sport, you may keep doing it as long as you feel comfortable. However, try to avoid making sudden, jerking movements because pregnancy hormones increase the risk of hurting your joints.

> ## *Cami's Story*
> In the first months of pregnancy, I went for a run several times a week. As my belly got bigger, it was hard to run as much. So I switched to taking a fast walk in the park. In the last month, my walks got slower. Then, when my legs started swelling, I went to the community pool. Swimming and water aerobics were great. I was able to exercise, and my feet were less swollen too.

Exercising the Pelvic Floor Muscles

The *pelvic floor* (or *perineal*) muscles surround your vagina. They support your uterus and other organs. During pregnancy, these muscles may sag and become weaker. Pelvic floor exercises help strengthen these muscles so you don't pee a little in your pants when you cough, sneeze, or laugh. Pelvic floor exercises also help reduce swelling and the heavy feeling around your vagina, may improve sex for you and your partner, and help prepare you for pushing out a baby.

To check the strength of your pelvic floor muscles, try stopping the flow of urine while you're peeing. If you can't stop the flow, it's a sign of weak muscles. Or you can insert two fingers (or your partner's penis) into your vagina and tighten the muscles. If they are weak, Kegel exercises will help. If your muscles are very tense, or if it hurts to have sex or it's painful or difficult to pee or poop, then pelvic floor bulging and relaxation will help.

Kegel Exercise (Pelvic Floor Contraction)
• Get in any position (sitting, standing, or lying down).
• Focus on the muscles around your *urethra* (where pee comes out) and vagina. Tighten those muscles as you would to stop the flow of pee. It should feel like you're lifting the pelvic floor. (Try not to tighten the muscles of your butt, thighs, or belly.)
• Hold the contraction as tightly as you can for a slow count of 10. (Don't hold your breath.)
• Repeat 10 times throughout the day.

Pelvic Floor Relaxation and Bulging
• Pee before doing this exercise. Then get in any position (sitting, standing, or lying down).
• Relax: Focus on the muscles around your urethra (where pee comes out) and vagina. Relax those muscles, imagine them letting go, melting, or becoming heavy.
• Bulge: Bear down gently with your pelvic floor muscles, as you do when having a bowel movement. (Don't bear down forcefully.)
• Hold for three to five seconds, then stop bearing down and relax.
• Do this once a day.

Have a Healthy Lifestyle

What else can you do to make your pregnancy as healthy as possible?

Get Enough Sleep and Rest

The amount of sleep you need may change as your pregnancy progresses. In early pregnancy, you may be sleepier than usual because of changes in your hormones. During the middle months, you may not need as much sleep. Later, as your baby grows, you'll use more energy to move around, and you'll be tired again. In late pregnancy, you'll probably wake up often during the night. See tips on page 49 if you're having trouble sleeping.

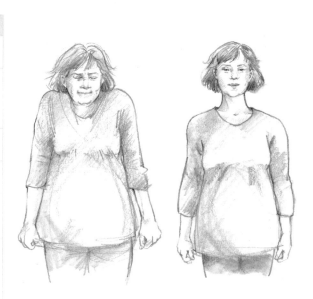

Relax to Reduce Stress

When you're upset or things feel really crazy, take some time for yourself. Learn how to calm your mind and reduce muscle tension.

The first step in learning how to relax is to notice how you feel when you are relaxed. For example, pay attention to how your mind and body feel when you're falling asleep. When you're drowsy, your muscles are loose, and your breathing is slow and even.

The next step is becoming aware of *muscle tension* (a tight feeling in your muscles) and learning how to relax.

Learning to Relax
When first learning to recognize muscle tension, practice in a quiet, calm place.
Make a tight fist with your right hand. Pay attention to how your arm and hand feel. Touch the muscles in your forearm with your other hand. Muscles are hard when they're tense.
Open your right hand and relax it. Notice how soft the muscles feel when you release the tension.
Next, raise your shoulders toward your ears. Notice how you feel when your shoulders are tense.
Lower your shoulders and relax. Release even more. Now really relax. Did you notice how you released more muscle tension when you became aware of it?
Continue to tighten and relax other muscles. Really notice how muscles feel when relaxed. Sometimes when you're stressed, your muscles tighten without your notice. Whenever you notice tension, relax and let go of it.
Take a deep breath and notice how relaxed you can feel.

Improve Stressful Relationships

Everyone has stressful relationships in some part of his or her life—with family, friends, or people at work. Most relationships have ups and downs. Pregnancy is a time to reduce contact or conflicts with people who cause you stress.

During pregnancy, you need someone in your life who cares for you and wants to help you. You need someone you trust and can talk to. Your partner, a family member, or a friend may be this person. If not, think of ways to work on those relationships or to make new connections, so you have the support you need.

It may help to meet other pregnant women by taking classes (prenatal exercise, yoga, or childbirth education) or by attending a pregnancy support group. Ask your caregiver about this. A social worker at the hospital can help you find support groups too.

Jenny's Story

When my sister, Luann, was pregnant, she had to move home because her boyfriend was so mean to her. We were afraid that he'd hurt her when he was drunk. Years ago, my mom kicked my dad out because he was hitting her. She wasn't going to let Luann go through that too. Mom helped Luann talk to the nurse about being abused. The nurse was real nice and told Luann where to go for help.

Kyle's not like that at all. He's a great guy. But some of his old friends weren't. Now that we've got a baby on the way, he's stopped hanging out with them, and I'm glad.

Getting Help from Others

What can your partner, family members, and friends do to help you during pregnancy?

- learn about pregnancy and how to help you during labor
- help you eat a healthy diet and avoid harmful behavior
- offer to help with household chores when you're tired
- enjoy having fun with you (seeing a movie, taking a walk, having a heart-to-heart talk, or laughing together)
- provide a peaceful, safe home (without fighting, hitting, pushing, or yelling)

Buckle Up: A Healthy Habit

You and your unborn baby are safer when you wear your seat belt in the car or on an airplane. Keep the belts tight across your shoulders and low on your hips. Buckle the belt below the bulge of your belly.

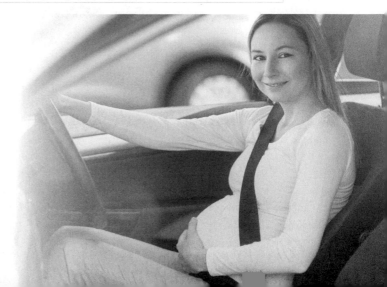

Avoid Harmful Substances

Everything you eat, drink, or breathe affects you. Some things can be harmful for your baby, while others are not. Your baby can handle exposure to some bad stuff, but reducing the following harmful substances as much as possible is best for your baby.

No Alcohol

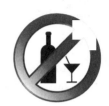

Alcohol is very bad for your baby. If you drink heavily during pregnancy (4 or more drinks a day), your baby may not grow well or ever learn normally because of brain damage. Even 2 drinks per day or binge drinking (more than 3 drinks) a few times during early pregnancy may cause mild learning and behavior problems for your child. Stop drinking when you're pregnant—the earlier the better.

No Tobacco

Cigarette smoke has many harmful substances, including tars, nicotine, carbon monoxide, and lead. Babies whose mothers smoke or are around secondhand smoke have lower-than-normal birth weights and may be born too early. Being around smoke during pregnancy or after birth increases a baby's risk of asthma and of dying of SIDS. Although e-cigarettes and snuff (smokeless tobacco) may be safer for adults than smoking is, they're not safe for baby. They contain nicotine, which may harm the baby's brain development and increases the chance the baby will have breathing problems after birth. Smoking substitutes, such as patches, gum, and nose sprays that contain nicotine, are also bad for baby.

If you use tobacco or nicotine products, stop or cut down as much as you can as soon as you can. Ask your caregiver about finding a program to help you stop smoking. If you live with people who smoke, ask them to smoke outside so you don't have to breathe it in.

No Marijuana

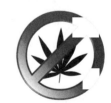

Don't consume marijuana (even if it's legal in your state). Whether you smoke or eat marijuana, it could affect your baby's brain development, causing lower scores on intelligence tests or problems with paying attention. If you use marijuana for medical reasons, ask your doctor if there is a better option during pregnancy.

No Drugs

Avoid using any illegal or dangerous drug, such as cocaine, heroin, or methamphetamines (meth). Also, avoid taking any prescription medications or over-the-counter medications unless your caregiver has prescribed them for you to take during pregnancy.

Illegal drugs and medications that are misused, can harm you and your baby in a variety of ways. They might cause *miscarriage* (death or delivery of a baby in early pregnancy), preterm birth, stillbirth, birth defects, or a very fussy baby. They might cause your placenta to separate too early or might cause a heart attack, stroke, or other health crises, as well as addiction. For your health and your baby's survival, it is best to avoid these drugs. For more information and for resources to help you quit, ask your caregiver or see http://www.marchofdimes.org/pregnancy/during -pregnancy-library.aspx.

Watch Out for Harmful Chemicals and Toxins

These substances may cause birth defects, preterm labor, or miscarriage:

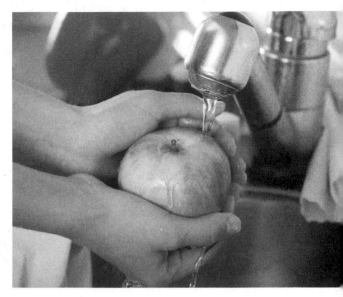

- products that kill insects or weeds (insecticides and herbicides)
- lead paint or asbestos in your home
- paint and paint thinners
- carbon monoxide (including exhaust from cars)
- chemicals like benzene and formaldehyde
- x-rays and other ionizing radiation
- some cleaning products

Here are some ideas on how to avoid harmful chemicals around your home or workplace:

- Wash fruits and vegetables.
- If using chemicals at home, wear protective gear, such as gloves or a mask. Or ask your partner or other household member to do that chore. For example, let someone else do any painting and stay away until the fumes are gone.
- If you or your partner work with chemicals or hazardous substances, take a shower and change clothes when you arrive home.
- In most cities in the United States and Canada, if your tap water comes from a city water supply, it's safe to drink. (If your city or water utility district has informed you that the water is contaminated, do not drink it.) If your water comes from a well, you may choose to drink bottled or filtered water.
- To learn more about chemicals and pregnancy, see http://www.mothertobaby.org.

Be Careful about Other Possible Hazards

Hot tubs and saunas. In early pregnancy, a high body temperature (over 100.4°F or 38°C) may cause birth defects in your baby. At other times in pregnancy, getting that hot may reduce blood flow to your uterus and baby. Therefore, avoid using hot tubs and saunas. You can take warm baths. If you begin to feel hot, get out of the tub or add some cool water.

Toxoplasmosis is an infection caused by a parasite spread through cat poop, raw meat, and unwashed vegetables. If you've already had it, your baby is safe because you can't get it again. However, if you catch this infection during pregnancy, it can cause deafness or other birth defects in your baby. Here's how to avoid getting it:

- Wash your hands after handling cats.
- Have someone else clean the litter box.
- Try not to work in a garden where cats may have pooped.
- Cook your meat well.
- Carefully wash all vegetables.

Follow Your Caregiver's Suggestions about Taking Medicines

Some medicines (such as antibiotics, insulin, and drugs for depression) *treat an illness*. If your caregiver orders a medicine, make sure to take it. Other medicines only *relieve symptoms*, such as pain, headache, runny nose, or cough. Look for other ways to deal with your pain or discomfort, such as using the home remedies suggested below.

A few common medicines that are harmless when you're not pregnant may cause problems when you're expecting a baby:

- **Drugs that reduce pain or fever**. Some pain relievers (such as aspirin, ibuprofen, and naproxen) increase the risk of bleeding in the mother and newborn baby. They also interfere with the start of labor. So don't take them when you're pregnant. Acetaminophen (Tylenol) may be used in pregnancy, but take only the suggested dose. Too much Tylenol can be harmful.

Home Remedies for a Headache

Instead of using medicine for a headache, try a warm bath, a massage, or tension-reducing exercises. Use the relaxation techniques suggested on pages 81–83. Hot packs or cold packs on the back of your neck, shoulders, or forehead may feel soothing. Try to get more sleep, and find time to rest during the day. Hunger can cause headaches, so don't miss a meal. Also, drink plenty of water.

- **Drugs to relieve symptoms of a cold**. Some cold medicines may be taken in pregnancy, while others should be avoided (see http://www.pcnguide.com). Talk with your caregiver. Because some cold medicines treat a wide range of symptoms and have several ingredients, always read the labels. You'll want to take only the specific drugs suggested by your caregiver.

Home Remedies for a Cold, Runny Nose, or Cough

These measures are safe in pregnancy:

- cool-mist vaporizer or a steamy shower
- saline nose spray or drops
- sleep and rest
- plenty of liquids

- drinking a mixture of honey and warm water
- additional doses of vitamin C
- hot soup, especially with added cayenne or other hot spices

---

- **Drugs to treat nausea and vomiting**. There aren't many safe over-the-counter drugs to help with vomiting. Try the suggestions on page 47 for reducing nausea. If they aren't enough and you're vomiting multiple times a day, talk to your caregiver about prescription drugs that may help.

Manage Common Pregnancy Discomforts

You'll probably have some of these normal (but irritating) discomforts during pregnancy. Try the following measures to help you cope. If you're worried, call your doctor or midwife for advice.

Nausea and Vomiting

It's common to feel sick to your stomach in the first months of pregnancy. This is sometimes called *morning sickness*, but it can happen anytime. You may feel like vomiting when you haven't eaten for several hours. Or your stomach may be upset when you smell strong odors.

To help prevent nausea and vomiting, try these suggestions:

- Eat a small snack when you first wake up. Protein is especially helpful.
- Eat 5 or 6 small meals each day to avoid having an empty stomach.
- Wear wristbands (Sea-Bands) that apply pressure on an *acupressure point* (a sensitive area) on your wrist to reduce seasickness and nausea.
- Eat foods high in vitamin B_6 or ask your caregiver about B_6 supplements.
- Eat foods that contain ginger (for example, fresh ginger, ginger ale, or ginger cookies) or peppermint.

Maria's Story

In the first 3 months of pregnancy, I felt sick to my stomach almost every morning. My friends and people at work all told me they'd had morning sickness. That made it a little easier to deal with. They also gave me great tips, such as putting some crackers and nuts by my bed so I could eat them as soon as I woke up. I ate half my lunch at 11 and the second half at 1:30. When I was queasy in the afternoon, I drank a glass of ginger ale. All those things helped.

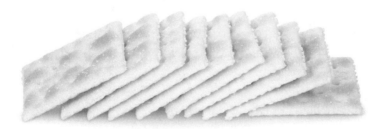

Heartburn

Heartburn (burping up stomach acid) is common in late pregnancy. It's caused by several factors. Pregnancy hormones relax the muscles at the top of your stomach and slow down the movement of food. Also, there's less room for food in your stomach as your baby grows. These suggestions may help:

- Avoid eating fatty foods and foods that produce gas or cause heartburn for you.
- Eat several small meals a day rather than a few large meals.
- Only drink a small amount of water with meals. (Drink plenty between meals.)
- Raise your head and shoulders with pillows, rather than lying flat in bed.
- Take antacids (acid reducers) or other drugs to control heartburn but only if suggested by your caregiver.

Constipation and Hemorrhoids

Constipation (hard bowel movements) is common in pregnancy. By preventing constipation, you can relieve another common problem during pregnancy: *hemorrhoids* (swollen veins in your rectum). The following suggestions may help:
- Drink plenty of water and other fluids.
- Eat high-fiber foods, such as fruits, vegetables, and whole-grain cereals and bread.
- Exercise (walk) each day.

If these measures don't help, talk to your caregiver about taking high-fiber products to soften your bowel movements. Don't take laxatives. Some iron pills cause constipation. If you're taking iron pills, change to a different kind.

Backaches

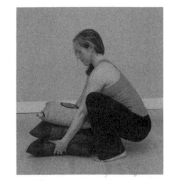

You may get a backache as your growing belly changes your shape. Try to prevent back pain by following these simple suggestions:
- Try to have good posture to ease strain in your back (see page 39).
- Be careful when lifting something heavy. Don't bend from the waist to pick it up. Bend your knees and hold it close to you as you stand up.
- Do exercises to strengthen your belly muscles and stretch your lower back muscles. (See the pelvic tilt exercise below.)

The following measures can help treat a backache:
- resting or sleeping more
- getting a massage or back rub
- using a cold pack or heating pad
- taking a warm bath or shower

How to Reduce Back Pain: The Pelvic Tilt Exercise

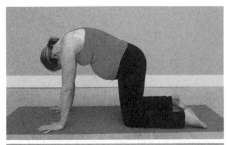

This exercise reduces lower back pain by strengthening the muscles in your belly.
1. Get on your hands and knees. Keep your back straight. (Do not sag.)
2. Tighten your belly muscles (this will tilt your pelvis forward and raise your lower back toward the ceiling).
3. Hold for a slow count of 5 as you breathe out.
4. Relax your belly and let your back go flat again as you slowly breathe in.
5. Repeat 10 times.

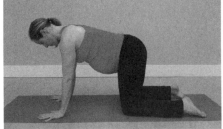

Swollen Legs and Feet

To reduce swelling in your feet and legs, try these comfort techniques:

- Drink plenty of water.
- Go swimming or soak your feet in cool water.
- Walk or move around. Avoid sitting or standing for a long period. If you have to be on your feet for a long time, shift your weight from foot to foot or march in place.
- When you sit, try to move your feet every 10 minutes by stretching and flexing your ankles. Don't cross your legs at the knees.
- Rock in a rocking chair.
- When resting, put your feet up.
- Ask your caregiver about wearing support stockings. To prevent swelling, put them on in the morning before your feet are swollen.

Leg and Foot Cramps

Cramps (severe pain) in the muscles of your lower legs or feet are common in late pregnancy. They usually happen when you're resting or asleep. To prevent cramps, avoid pointing your toes, standing on tiptoes, and curling your toes. Also, make sure there's plenty of calcium and magnesium in your diet and drink plenty of water during the day to help prevent muscle cramps at night.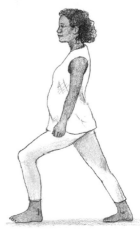

To relieve a muscle cramp, slowly stretch the painful muscle:

- For a cramp in your calf, stand with your weight on the cramped leg. Keep your leg straight and your heel on the floor. Step forward with your other leg and bend that knee. Lean forward to stretch the calf muscle of the straight leg.
- For a cramp in your foot, pull your toes up toward your shin. This stretches your toes and the bottom of your foot.

Trouble Sleeping

It's common to have trouble getting a good night's sleep, especially in late pregnancy. If you can find time to exercise or take a walk during the day, it may help you sleep better at night. Don't exercise shortly before bedtime, as this can wake you up.

So try to budget about 9 hours for sleep each night. This may mean that you have to go to bed earlier or stay in bed later to get enough sleep. When you're tired during the day, try to take a nap or sit down to rest. Try these suggestions at bedtime:

- Take a warm bath.
- Drink a glass of warm milk.
- Have a massage.
- Listen to soothing music.

If you find yourself awake in the middle of the night, try using the relaxation techniques described on pages 81–83. Don't turn on a screen and start reading social media.

CHAPTER 5

Preparing for Birth

What should you do to get ready for labor and birth? This chapter suggests some things to do before your baby is born:

- Learn more about childbirth and what choices you will have.
- Make a plan about what you want during labor.
- See the birthing rooms at your hospital or birth center.
- Get ready for the hospital or birth center by filling out forms and packing your bag.

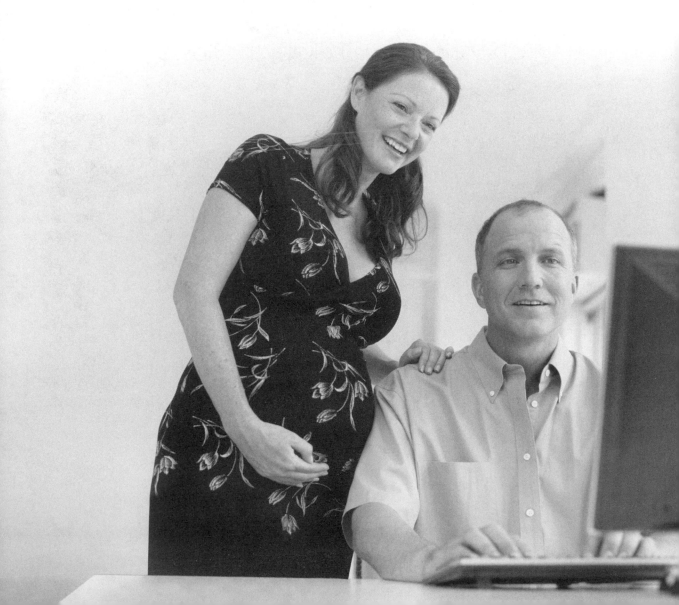

What Choices Do You Have?

You'll be asked to make some choices about your care during childbirth. It helps to have good information about your options.

Some women search online for information, but not everything you find online is up to date, or true, or common practice where you live. Some women ask other women about labor. This is often helpful, but some birth stories may be upsetting, or unusual, or may be very different from what you might experience.

Better sources of information include childbirth classes and your caregiver. They can give you up-to-date information about how women are cared for at your birthplace and can tell you about many different birth experiences and what is most likely for you. Learning about your choices helps you make realistic plans for your baby's birth.

Choosing Your Childbirth Classes

Some hospitals, community groups, and prenatal clinics offer classes. The best classes include information about the following things:

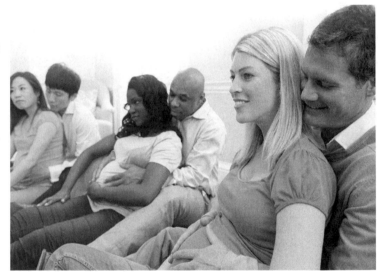

- childbirth (what to expect and what you can do)
- choices that are available to you and your *birth partner* (the person with you during labor and birth)
- ways of handling labor pain (you may practice breathing and comfort techniques)
- caring for your baby and your-self after birth
- breastfeeding your baby

Classes also give you time to ask questions and a chance to meet other people who are having babies.

To learn where to go for classes, talk with your caregiver and friends. Since classes may fill up early, try to sign up before the sixth month of your pregnancy. There are fees for classes. Medicaid may pay for them in some states.

John's Story

I was glad that Maria and I decided to take childbirth classes. Before class, I was afraid I'd be useless during labor. But in class, we learned lots of things I can do to help. The videos also showed us what it would be like in the hospital. They made labor and birth seem less like a big scary unknown. I learned how to help with breastfeeding, and I didn't even know I needed to learn that.

Planning Your Baby's Birth

Getting ready for childbirth is like getting ready for any other big event in your life: You make plans. If you prepare for it, you'll know what to expect and will feel more in control. Begin preparing for the birth by thinking about things that are important to you. Then make a list of your needs and wishes. This is called a *birth plan*.

Jenny's Story

I really hate needles. In my birth plan, I said that I didn't want any needles if I could help it. But I said that if I do need one, I need my mom or Kyle to hold my hand and talk me through it, and I need to know exactly when they're going to put the needle in.

My sister gave me some ideas about what else to ask. Luann loved the bathtub, and it made her labor go faster. Kyle and I talked a lot about other coping techniques we learned in class. I'm hoping not to use pain medications, so I wrote in my birth plan some ways that the nurse, Mom, and Kyle can help me. Having a plan helped me feel prepared.

The Birth Plan

A birth plan is a letter to your caregivers (doctors, midwives, and nurses) describing how you'd like to be cared for. Here are some reasons to write one:

- It encourages you to think about what you need and want.
- It helps you learn about your choices.
- It lets your caregivers know what's most important to you and why.
- It helps you work with your birth partners in planning the best birth experience possible.

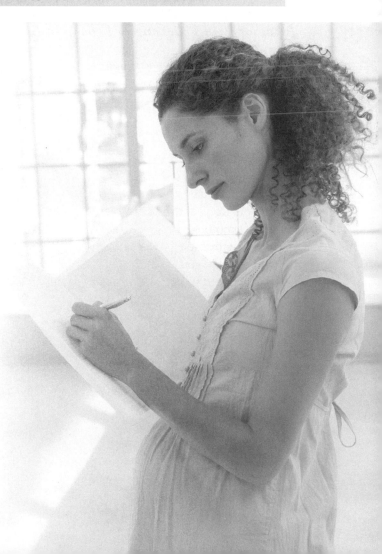

It's a good idea to prepare your birth plan over several weeks. It takes time to find out about your choices.

When preparing a birth plan, you and your caregivers work together to make a general plan for a normal birth without medical problems. You can also plan for any problems that may come up.

What Do You Put in Your Birth Plan?

For each of the six sections below, write a few sentences to build your birth plan.

Information You Want Staff to Know about You

Share a little about yourself:
- Who will be with you during labor? Your partner? A friend? A family member? A doula? (See page 88 for information about doulas.)
- Who will be helping you to parent this baby?
- If you have other children, share a little about their births.
- Do you have religious or cultural customs that may affect your labor and birth?
- Do you need a translator?

Important Issues, Fears, or Concerns You May Have

If you have concerns, such as a fear of needles, past medical problems, or concerns about modesty or other issues, share this in your birth plan. That helps your nurses to support you better.

Your Plans for Pain Relief during Labor and Birth

- How do you plan to cope with labor? Do you prefer relaxation and breathing techniques? Walking? Using a birth ball? Taking a tub bath? (See pages 81–86 for more information.)
- When labor becomes hard for you, do you want to be encouraged to keep trying to cope with labor? Or do you want to be offered pain medication? What kind of pain medicine would you want (see pages 94–96)?

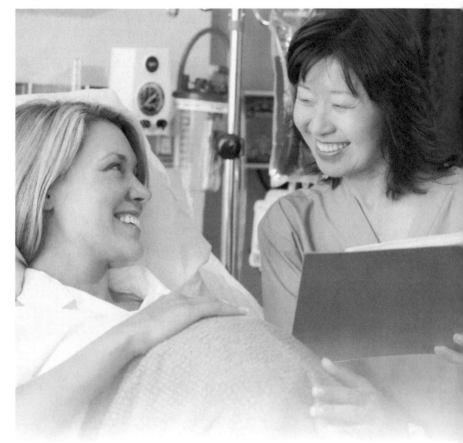

Your Plans for Medical Care and Procedures during Normal Labor and Birth

- Do you have strong feelings about having (or not having) these common medical practices and procedures:
    - IV fluids (see page 71)
    - staying in bed with constant electronic fetal monitoring (EFM) (see page 70)
    - choose a birthing position (see page 75)
    - episiotomy (see page 106)
- How would you like your caregiver and nurse to care for you during labor? Would you like the staff to stay in your room to comfort you? Would you like to be alone with your birth partner as much as possible?

Your Plans for When Labor Doesn't Go as Expected

- If there are medical reasons to induce labor, would you prefer to try self-help methods to start labor, or medical induction methods (see pages 100–101)?
- What do you want to do if labor is long and slow (see pages 104–106)?
- What are your plans if a cesarean birth is needed (see pages 107–111)?
- What would you like to happen if your baby has a health problem?

Your Plans for Caring for Yourself and Your Baby after Birth

- How will you feed your baby? Breastfeeding or formula feeding (see chapter 10)?
- If your baby is male, do you want him to be circumcised?
- Do you have any concerns or thoughts about the normal newborn tests or procedures (see page 77)?
- Do you need certain foods or care because of customs of your family, religion, or native culture?
- Do you have any needs after going home? Help with buying food? Help getting medical care for you or your baby?

See pages 58–59 for a blank birth plan. You can copy it and use it for your own birth plan.

Cami's Story

I had hoped to have a birth without a lot of medications or interventions. But after I developed gestational hypertension, I asked my doctor how that would change my birth plan. She said it was more likely we would need to induce labor. She said Pitocin can make the contractions hurt more, so I decided I might use an epidural. We also talked about writing a birth plan for a cesarean just in case. I asked if I would be able to have my baby skin-to-skin with me and breastfeed while the cesarean was being finished, and she said that we would have to ask the anesthesiologist. I didn't want to think about having a cesarean, but it helped to have talked about my options.

Taking a Tour of Your Hospital or Birth Center

A good way to find out about your birthplace's rules and procedures (called routines) is to take a tour. You'll be shown the birthing rooms, postpartum rooms, and the family waiting area. The tour guide will discuss typical routines and answer any questions you have. To schedule a tour, call your birthplace or look on their website.

Registering at the Hospital or Birth Center

You may be asked to fill out admission forms before you are in labor so you have time to think about them and ask questions about anything you don't understand. The forms may include a general consent form, which allows the staff to care for you. In the hospital, you may be asked to sign other forms for procedures, such as epidural anesthesia or cesarean birth.

Note to Fathers and Partners

Plan to attend childbirth classes and go on the birthplace tour with your partner. Learning more about the birth process will help you feel more confident in your ability to provide support during labor and birth. Also, work with your partner on creating the birth plan. People in labor tend to cope best if all they have to focus on is dealing with the pain. Having you there to answer questions from caregivers, ask questions about procedures, and make informed choices will allow your partner to relax and respond to instincts for how to cope.

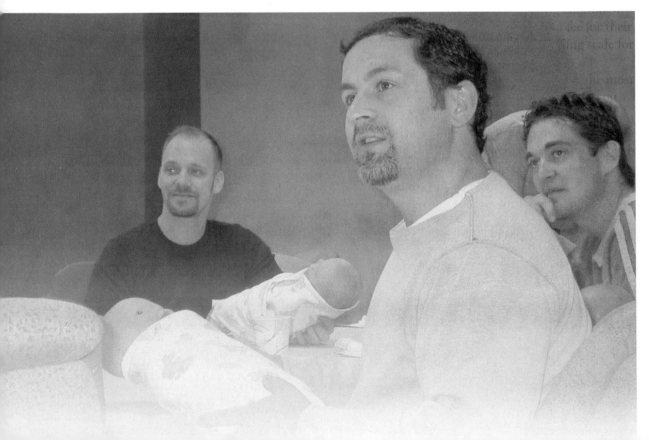

Packing Your Bag for the Hospital or Birth Center

Even though you'll be in the hospital or birth center for only a short time, you'll be happier if you have some of these personal items:

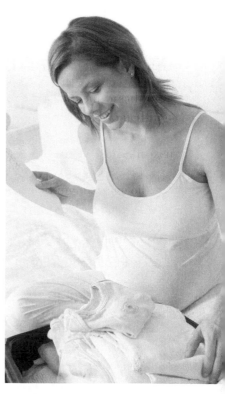

- this book
- hairband, headband, or barrette (to keep your hair off your face)
- lip gloss or balm
- toothbrushes (for you and your partner) and toothpaste
- personal comfort items (pillow from home, pictures, warm or cold packs, and so on)
- warm socks
- hot water bottle (or fill a sock with uncooked rice, tie off the open end, and heat it in a microwave for 3 to 5 minutes)
- nightgown (if you don't want to wear a hospital gown during labor)
- pajamas or a nightgown that opens easily for breastfeeding
- snacks for your partner
- camera or video camera (check the birthplace's policies on recording births)
- phone numbers of people to call after the birth (check the birthplace's policy on cell phone use)
- CD or MP3 player of relaxing music (ask about available equipment)
- robe and slippers (or use ones from the hospital)
- hairbrush, makeup, shampoo, or other toiletries
- nursing bra
- loose-fitting clothes (probably your maternity clothes) to wear when going home
- clothes for the baby, including an undershirt or "onesie" (one-piece body suit), diapers (cloth ones with waterproof cover or disposable diapers), one-piece footed outfit, large lightweight blankets, warm (outside) blanket, and hat
- car seat, already installed in your car (see page 168)

If you'll be giving birth at a birth center, you'll need most of these same items even though your stay will be shorter. If you're planning a home birth, ask your midwife or doctor about supplies and special preparations that you'll need in your home.

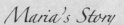

Maria's Story

After the classes, we were feeling much more prepared for labor. But it seemed like a good idea to have an extra person around who had more experience than John or I did. So we wanted to hire a doula. For our baby shower, we asked for money to cover that. All the things we needed for baby we were able to get at consignment stores or as hand-me-downs from friends and family. We decided that having support for a great birth was more important than having more baby clothes or rattles.

Birth Plan

Name_____ Due date_____

Doctor's or midwife's name _____

Birth setting (name of hospital or birth center) _____

_____

This is my plan for labor and birth.
I want to let you know what is important to me.
I know that this plan may have to change if problems come up.
Thank you for your help and support.

Introducing myself:

Some helpful information about me: _____

_____

_____

Some information about my birth partner(s): _____

_____

_____

Important issues, fears, and concerns of mine: _____

_____

_____

My wishes for pain relief and comfort during labor and birth:_____

_____

_____

_____

My wishes for medical care and procedures with normal labor and birth: _____

_____

_____

_____

My wishes if labor doesn't go as expected:

With a long, slow labor: _____

_____

_____

If my baby needs a cesarean birth: _____

_____

_____

If my baby has health problems: _____

_____

_____

My wishes for caring for my baby and myself after the birth:

Feeding my baby: Breast milk ☐   Formula ☐

My thoughts about baby care in the hospital / birth center: _____

_____

_____

Requests for special care or foods: _____

_____

I want to learn about these things while in the hospital / birth center: _____

_____

_____

_____

We need help with these things after we go home: _____

_____

_____

_____

CHAPTER 6
Having Your Baby: Labor and Birth

If you're having your first baby, you probably have a lot of questions about what to expect during labor and birth. In this chapter, find out what is going on inside of you during labor and what words your caregivers will use to talk about that process. We'll also discuss how you'll feel, what your partner can do to help, and what your caregivers can do for you during labor.

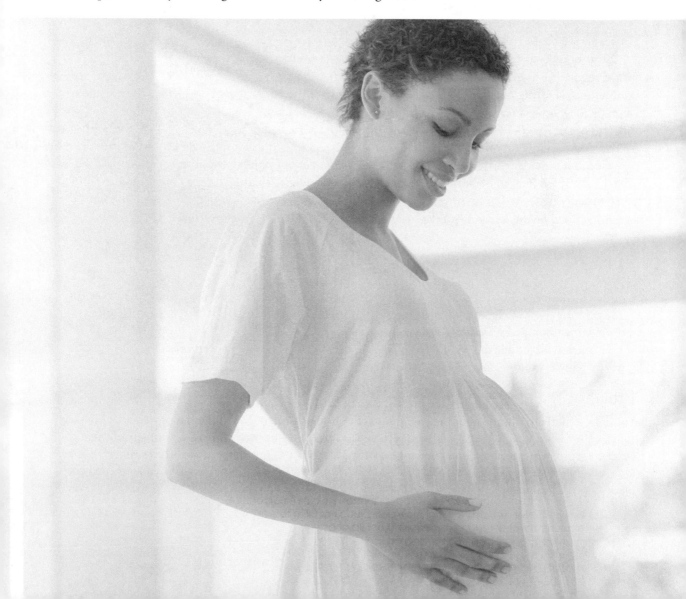

Late Pregnancy: How Labor Begins

In the final weeks of pregnancy, both you and your baby are preparing for birth. You start to make breast milk (*colostrum*). Your
baby gets antibodies from you (these protect her from infections
after she is born). Her brain grows bigger and smarter. Her lungs
mature so that she will be able to breathe on her own after birth.

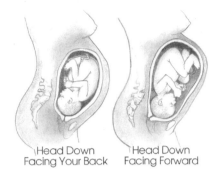

Head Down
Facing Your Back

Head Down
Facing Forward

Your baby moves into position for labor. During most of
pregnancy, your baby moves around a lot your uterus. By week 33
to 35, most babies get into a head-down position with their face
toward the mother's front or back. This means that his head will
come out first when he's born. It's possible for a baby's bottom or
feet to be down low, but this is rare (only 3–4% of babies). This
is called a *breech presentation*. Most breech babies are delivered by
cesarean. (See pages 107–111 for more on cesarean.)

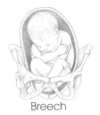

Breech

Your body is also preparing for labor. Your uterus becomes
sensitive to a hormone called *oxytocin*, and you will have more
contractions. During pregnancy, your cervix is firm. At the end
of pregnancy, other hormones cause it to *ripen* (soften). Then it's
ready to open. Ripening may begin in the last weeks of pregnancy or just a few days before labor begins.
You can't see your cervix from the outside, but your caregiver can feel it during a vaginal exam.

Hormones made by the mother and baby set off a chain of events that start labor, usually at the
time the baby is ready to be born and the mother is ready to give birth. At some point, you'll go into
labor (usually between 2 weeks before and 2 weeks after your due date). If you experience the signs of
labor described below *before* 37 weeks, you may be in preterm labor. To learn more, see page 30.

Stages of Labor

Childbirth (labor and birth) may take anywhere from a few hours to a few days. You can't know for
sure how long it will take. It's different for every woman. Also, it's usually different each time any
individual woman gives birth.

Caregivers describe labor as a series of stages, which describe how the cervix is changing, and
how the baby is moving toward birth.

Prelabor

You may experience contractions before labor really begins. (See page 65 to learn more about contractions.) They help ripen and *efface* the cervix (make it softer and thinner). *Effacement* can be measured in
percentages or centimeters: 0% effaced means that the cervix has not thinned at all (it's still 4 centimeters
long, about 1½ inches). During labor, it will reach 100% effaced, which means that it has thinned completely until it's almost paper-thin. Because prelabor contractions don't usually *dilate* (open) the cervix,
this is sometimes called "false labor." It may last for a few hours or a few days.

First Stage

Your contractions get stronger and more regular. They push the baby down onto your cervix. This opens the cervix. When the cervix is opened only the width of a fingertip, it's called 1 centimeter dilated. When the cervix is fully open, it's about 10 centimeters dilated. It may seem hard to imagine that it opens that far, but remember: It's exactly what your body is designed to do during labor.

The contractions are also moving your baby downward. This is called *descent*. Your baby has to turn as she moves down the birth canal. This allows her head to fit through your pelvis. This is called *rotation*.

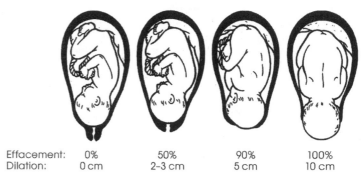

| Effacement: | 0% | 50% | 90% | 100% |
| Dilation: | 0 cm | 2–3 cm | 5 cm | 10 cm |

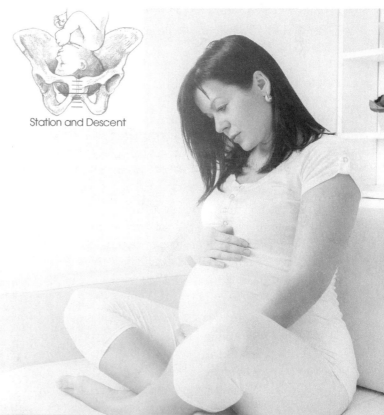

Station and Descent

Second Stage

Contractions press your baby through the cervix, out of your uterus into your vagina (birth canal). Then you push until your baby is born.

Third Stage

These contractions work to push out the placenta.

Fourth Stage

This refers to the first few hours after birth. It's also called *recovery*.

Cami's Story

When I was pregnant, all my friends who had babies wanted to tell me what labor felt like. One said, "At first, it's hard to tell if it's labor or not. I thought I was in labor 3 or 4 times, but the contractions would just go away. Then the day my son was born, they didn't quit. They just kept coming and coming, and then I knew it was real labor."

Another friend said, "My bag of waters broke all at once—in our bed! I felt like I was peeing in my pants and couldn't stop. Then the contractions came hard and fast. No prelabor for me."

Some of my friends had really short labors, and some had really long labors. Some felt really powerful after getting through it without drugs, and others told me that there was no way they could have done it without the epidural. Since it seems like I can't predict what will happen, Chris and I have talked a lot in advance about what I would want to do if different things come up.

How Do You Know You're in Labor?

The following signs (or *physical symptoms*) will help you figure out if you're in labor.

Possible Signs of Labor

Any of the following can happen in the days or weeks before labor begins:

- lower backache that may come and go and make it hard to sit still
- cramps (like menstrual cramps) in your lower belly
- several soft bowel movements or diarrhea-like BMs, or upset stomach
- sudden burst of energy focused on getting ready for the baby (called the *nesting urge*)

Prelabor Signs

These are signs that your cervix is starting to change and labor may begin in a few hours or a few days:

- Prelabor contractions. They may come and go, or may develop into a pattern where contractions are several minutes apart. But they do not progress (do not get longer or stronger or closer together).
- Increased vaginal mucus. It may be mixed with a little blood (called *bloody show*).
- A small amount of water leaking from your vagina. (This *may* be your bag of waters breaking.)

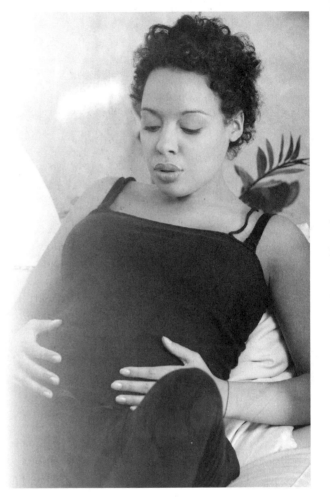

Positive Signs of Labor

These are the clearest signs that labor has started:

- You see or feel a gush of water from your vagina caused by the bag of waters breaking.
- Your contractions get longer, stronger, and closer together as time goes on. These are called *progressing contractions.*
- To test whether you are having progressing contractions, try drinking water or changing your activity. Contractions may slow or stop. But if they continue to get longer, stronger, and closer together, it's likely to be true labor.

Jenny's Story

In the beginning, labor contractions felt like big muscle cramps in my belly. You know how your arm muscles start to ache when you're holding something heavy for a long time? That's what early labor felt like for me. At the time, I thought it might feel like that until the baby was born. I was wrong.

What Do Labor Contractions Feel Like?

By the end of pregnancy, your uterus is the largest and strongest muscle in your body. When it contracts (tightens), it hardens and bulges like any other muscle. See the box below to learn how to feel for a contraction.

Contractions come and go during labor. Each contraction is like a wave: It's weak in the beginning, it builds to a peak, and then it gradually goes away. Between contractions, your uterus rests. As labor goes on, these rest periods get shorter, and the contractions get longer and stronger. Early in labor, contractions may feel like a dull lower backache or menstrual cramps. Some women describe them as a tightening or feeling of their belly muscles pulling inward. They come and go. These early contractions are usually (though not always) short and mild. As labor advances, you'll feel the contractions in your belly or in your lower back or both. Many women feel the pain begin in the back and come around to the front. If your contractions keep coming but last less than 30 seconds, if they're not very strong, and if they don't get closer together, you're still in prelabor or entering early labor. In true labor, your contractions will become stronger, longer, and/or closer together. For example, your labor might begin with contractions that are a little uncomfortable, 30 seconds long, and 15 minutes apart. Later, they're painful, 45 seconds long, and 7 minutes apart.

Checking for Contractions
Pee, then drink 2 big glasses of water
Sit with your feet up and relax
Place your fingertips on your belly at the top of your uterus (the fundus). When you feel the uterus get tight, press gently but firmly. If the fundus feels like your forehead and you can't indent it (push it in), that's a strong contraction. (If you're full-term, this contraction will probably hurt. But if these are preterm contractions, they may be this strong but not hurt.) If it feels like your nose or chin, that's a moderate contraction. If it feels like your cheek when you puff it out, that's a mild contraction and less likely to be true labor.
Press your fingers in multiple places. Generally, if your whole uterus is tight, it's a contraction, but if only one spot is firm, that may just be your baby pushing against your belly.
Count the contractions for 1 hour.

Timing Labor Contractions

Timing your contractions can help you decide if you're truly in labor. You need to know 3 main terms to describe your contractions:

1. *Length* (how long a contraction lasts, in seconds)
2. *Frequency* (how often the contractions are coming—for example, every 5 minutes)
3. *Intensity* (how strong the contractions feel)

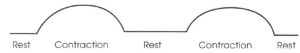

Rest   Contraction   Rest   Contraction   Rest

There are several websites and mobile apps you can use to time your contractions. Or you can use this clock, pencil, and paper method.

1. When a contraction begins, write down the time.
2. When the contraction ends, figure out the number of seconds from the beginning of the contraction until the end. This is the *length* of the contraction.

3. To find out the *frequency*, time 5 or 6 contractions in a row. Figure out the number of minutes from the beginning of 1 contraction to the beginning of the next.

4. To find out the strength or *intensity* of the contractions, compare the ones you're having now with the ones you had an hour ago. Do they seem stronger now? Are they more painful? If so, they're more intense.

Early Labor Record (sample)			
Contractions on April 29			
Time	**Length**	**Frequency**	**Comments**
Starting time	How many seconds long?	How many minutes since the beginning of the last one?	Intensity of contractions, food eaten, breathing level, bloody show, status of membranes, other events
1:54 am	40 seconds	_	Bloody show started at 6 pm
2:03 am	45 seconds	9 minutes	Can't sleep
2:10 am	45 seconds	7 minutes	Loose BM, backache
2:17 am	50 seconds	7 minutes	Stronger!

When to Call Your Caregiver

During the last month of your pregnancy, ask your caregiver for advice about when you should call and whom you should call. You may be told to call the hospital birthing unit (especially at night). Or you may be told to call your midwife or doctor directly. Here are some general guidelines:

- Call when your bag of waters breaks.
- Once you have progressing contractions (they're getting longer, stronger, and closer together), use the *4-1-1 Rule.* Call when contractions are less than 4 minutes apart, at least 1 minute long, and you've had this pattern for 1 hour or more. At this point, it's also usually difficult for you to talk or walk during a contraction, because coping with the contraction takes all your attention.
- If you've had a baby before, your caregiver may tell you not to wait that 1 hour. He or she may tell you to call as soon as you have contractions that are 4 minutes apart and 1 minute long.
- Your caregiver may tell you to call earlier if you have a medical problem or if you live far away.
- Call if you're anxious or have questions, even if you're not sure you're in labor. Make sure you have someone to drive you to the hospital day or night. Keep phone numbers handy. If you don't know anyone, choose a cab company and write down the number ahead of time or program it into your phone. Keep enough cash in your purse or have your taxi voucher ready.

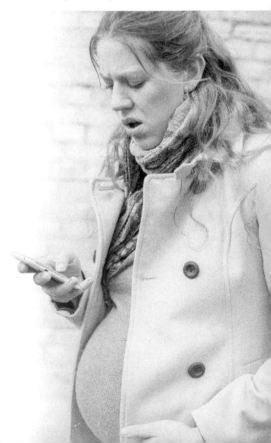

Getting through the First Stage of Labor

The first stage of labor is divided into three phases (parts):

1. *Early labor.* This is the longest phase, but contractions are usually short and not very painful.
2. *Active labor.* Contractions are harder (more intense).
3. *Transition.* This is the shortest phase, but contractions are most intense.

Your feelings will change as you go from 1 phase to another. Also, your coping skills will need to change as you move through each phase. In a childbirth class, you would practice many of these skills. This chapter and the Road Map of Labor (see pages 196–197) will help to remind you of which coping skills are helpful in each phase.

Early Labor

In the early phase of labor, this is what contractions usually look like:

*   They come every 6–20 minutes. (They start as much as 20 minutes apart and get closer together as time goes on until they're about 6 minutes apart.)
*   They last 20–60 seconds. (They may start out as short as 20 seconds. They become longer until they last about 60 seconds.)
*   They feel like strong menstrual cramps or mild pain in your belly and/or lower back.
*   They cause bloody show to pass from your vagina.

During early labor, your cervix thins out and opens to 4 or 5 centimeters. You won't know this without a vaginal exam, but if you see the symptoms above, they're generally a good sign of cervical change.

You'll probably spend most of early labor at home doing normal activities. You'll rest if it's nighttime and keep busy if it's daytime. Try not to do too much since you'll need plenty of energy for labor.

You'll probably feel excited and a bit nervous. Most likely, you'll want a family member or a friend with you.

What to Do in Early Labor

*   Pack your bag (or prepare your home if you're planning a home birth).
*   Go for a walk, listen to music, or watch a movie.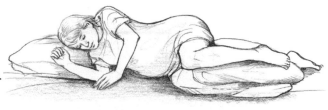
*   Eat foods and drink beverages that are easy to digest, such as noodle soup, fruit, yogurt, pasta, toast, and herbal tea. Fatty foods aren't good at this time. They may upset your stomach.
*   Do a fun project at home to focus on. For example, bake a cake. This will help distract you from worrying too much about labor.
*   If you're tired, try to rest. Have someone give you a back rub.
*   Use comfort techniques to relax your muscles and calm your mind (see pages 81–83).
*   Take a long shower (but *not* a long bath as it could slow labor progress at this time).
*   The key focus in early labor is *relaxation*. Do anything that helps to relax you. Breathe. Focus on something other than your worries. Keep the environment safe and soothing and try to enjoy this time.

Getting into Active Labor

When the contractions become painful and you can't walk or talk during a contraction, it's time to use your coping skills (see pages 87–90). Use slow breathing. Try to stay relaxed, even limp, during the intense contractions. Keep your mind on calming thoughts, music, or pictures. It may help to rock or sway in one of the positions shown on the Road Map. Between contractions, go back to whatever you were doing before the contraction.

Start working with your partner so he or she knows how to help you during the rest of your labor. Some people have an experienced woman (*birth doula*) come to their home to help them with early contractions.

There is a period between early labor and active labor where contractions get much closer together and much more painful, but labor progress may go much slower than you wished between 4 and 6 centimeters of dilation. Don't be discouraged if you arrive at the hospital in what feels like hard active labor, and they tell you your cervix shows you are still in early labor. Let your body do the hard work it needs to do, and soon the cervix will start to change more.

Maria's Story

I knew I was in labor when I couldn't walk or talk through a contraction. It really hurt. When a contraction started, I had to stop everything except my special breathing and rocking back and forth. I needed that rhythm. The good thing about labor is that every contraction goes away, so you get a little break before the next one. John would remind me to relax as much as I could during those breaks to save my energy.

Active Labor

Most women go to the hospital or birth center when they enter the active phase of labor. (See page 66 for when to call.) In active labor, contractions continue to become longer, stronger, and closer together. This is what you can expect contractions to look like in this phase:

*   last 60 seconds or longer
*   feel intense and painful
*   come every 3–5 minutes

During this phase, labor speeds up, and your cervix usually dilates faster than before. During active labor, the cervix dilates from 5 or 6 cm to 8 cm.

In active labor, you become serious, quiet, and focused on your contractions. Earlier, your partner's jokes and talk were fun; now you can't listen. You don't want people asking you questions or talking to you during contractions. You may feel tired. Many people in labor feel like they can't keep going.

The key for coping with active labor is to remember *rhythm is everything*. You may find yourself rocking in rhythm, breathing in rhythm, and so on. When we're working well with our bodies, we have rhythm. (Think about when you're hammering a nail, or stirring cake batter, or jumping rope. You need rhythm to make it work.) If you find a rhythm that works for you, your partner should support it. For example, if you are breathing in rhythm, your partner can stroke your arm in the same rhythm. It may be hard for you to keep the rhythm during the most painful part of the contraction. If your partner helps you hold that rhythm, that will help you feel like you can handle the contraction better.

What to Do in Active Labor

- Breathe in a rhythm during contractions.
- Relax between contractions.
- Move around. Try changing positions to get more comfortable (walking, standing, leaning on your partner or the bed, or rocking in a rocking chair).
- Move, rock, or sway in rhythm (like slow dancing).
- Have your partner massage or stroke you in rhythm with your breathing.
- Sit on or lean over a birth ball.
- Get into a bathtub or take a shower.
- Drink water or suck on ice chips.
- Go to the bathroom and empty your bladder about once an hour.
- Rest when needed.
- Listen to music.
- Use warm or cold packs.
- Remember that the pain of contractions is normal. It's not harmful.

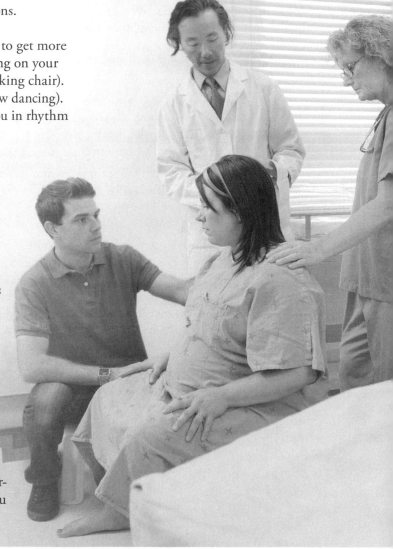

Your partner should move in closer now. He or she should remain calm and share your serious mood. Your partner can help you stay with your breathing patterns and find comfortable positions. Your partner can also try softly touching or stroking you. What you need now is someone to help you feel loved. If you feel frightened or worried, you will have more pain because of stress hormones. If you feel safe, secure, and loved, you will release different hormones, which help you feel less pain and help labor to go faster.

Maria's Story

I got awfully tired during labor. I worried that getting so little sleep meant that I wouldn't be able to cope with the pain. John was having trouble staying awake too. Our doula said, "This would be a great time for a nice, deep warm bath. It'll help you relax. And John can nap while I sit with you so he has energy later on." I loved the warm water. Katie closed the door, put on quiet music, and dimmed the lights. Then she sat near me and helped me relax when contractions came. I actually slept a little in the tub.

Hospital Routines

When you give birth in a hospital, the nurses, doctors, and midwives use tests and procedures to check your progress and make sure you and your baby are doing well. These common medical procedures are called *routines* because they're given to almost every woman who gives birth at that hospital.

Checking on the Baby

One way to check on the baby's health is to count the heartbeats of the baby (*fetus*) when the mother is having a contraction and right after the contraction is over. This is called *fetal monitoring*. If the baby's heart rate looks fine, it's a good sign that the baby is doing well. If the heart rate isn't acting as expected, it doesn't necessarily mean there's something wrong. However, it does mean caregivers will want to monitor more closely, because it can sometimes mean that the baby isn't getting enough oxygen from the placenta.

There are 3 ways to monitor the heart rate:

1. The nurse listens to the fetal heartbeats by holding a *Doppler* (an ultrasound stethoscope like the one used during your prenatal visits) on your belly for about a minute. The heart rate is counted every 15–30 minutes during labor (and more often during the second stage). If you are giving birth at home or at a birth center, this is how your baby's heart rate will be monitored.

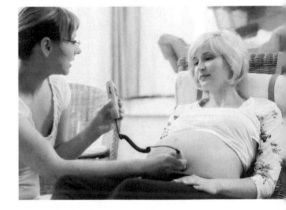

2. With *external electronic fetal monitoring (EFM)*, the nurse places 2 pieces of equipment (sensors) on your belly and holds them in place with elastic bands. One keeps track of contractions. The other measures the baby's heart rate. Both are connected to a machine that shows the information on a screen and makes a printed record. This is typically done for 15 minutes of each hour. If you are at high risk of problems, you might have continuous EFM, where the monitor is on at all times. Many hospitals have wireless monitoring, which allows you to move around or take a bath. Ask for it if it's not offered to you.

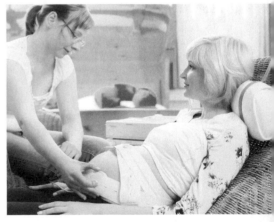

3. *Internal EFM* may be used if the other methods have shown that your baby might be having a problem. With internal EFM, 2 pieces of equipment are inserted through your vagina into your uterus. One is attached to the baby's head to measure the baby's heart rate. The other measures how strong the contractions are.

A Reminder
Remember that you can always ask for more information about any procedure before agreeing to have it done. Sometimes the stress of being in the hospital makes it hard to understand what your caregivers are telling you about your care. If you don't understand the first answer, ask again. It's your right to know what's happening to you. Ask these key questions: • **Benefits:** Why do you recommend this procedure? • **Risks:** Are there any reasons not to do it? • **Options:** Is there anything else I could try? • **Timing:** Is this an emergency? How quickly do I need to make a decision?

Checking on the Mother

Throughout labor, the nurse checks many signs that tell about your health and how fast your labor is going.

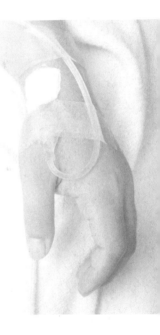

- The nurse watches and records your blood pressure, temperature, pulse (heart rate), urine output (how much you're peeing), and fluid intake (how much you're drinking).
- Vaginal exams help your nurse or caregiver check your labor progress (whether your cervix is thinning and opening and your baby is moving down).
- Your nurse or midwife will check the frequency and intensity of your contractions by either feeling your belly or using EFM.

Intravenous (IV) Fluids

IV fluid is water mixed with minerals given to you through a tube inserted in a vein (blood vessel below your skin) in your arm or hand. The fluid drips through the tube from an IV bag that hangs from a stand near the bed. An IV makes sure your body has enough fluids. (If you are in good health, you may not need an IV. You can drink water or juice instead.) An IV is also a good way to give you medicine quickly if you need it.

Learn more about hospital routines at http://www.lamaze.org/MedicalInterventions.

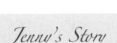

Jenny's Story

I'd planned to not use drugs, but in labor, I didn't think I could do it. It was so hard. I cried. I said, "I hate this! Get me drugs!" My mom and Kyle never said yes or no. They just kept telling me, "You're doing so well—keep that rhythm." So I just kept doing the same things. Every contraction, I rocked on a birth ball, stared at a picture of my cat, and did the breathing. I moaned a lot too. I hated labor, but after a while I knew I could do it. I stopped asking for drugs and kept my mind on the rhythm and my mom's voice.

Transition

This phase is usually the most difficult part of labor, but it's the shortest. For a first-time mother, transition is usually about 1 hour long. For mothers having a second baby, it may be even shorter. These contractions aren't much more painful than those in the active phase, but they seem harder because they're longer and closer together. During this phase, this is what you can expect your contractions to do:

- come every 2–3 minutes
- last 1–2 minutes (sometimes before one goes away, another one starts)
- feel very strong because the time is so short between them (30–90 seconds)
- dilate your cervix to 10 centimeters

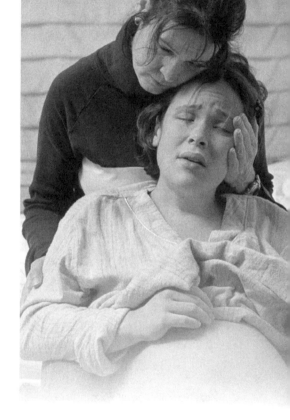

You may have some or all of these normal signs of transition:

- bag of waters breaking (if it hasn't already) and more bloody show
- nausea, vomiting, or hiccups
- shaking of your legs or your whole body
- changing back and forth between feeling cold and shivering and feeling hot and sweaty
- pressure in your vagina and rectum that makes you want to grunt or strain hard, as if you're having a bowel movement (however, it may be too early for you to push)

Strong emotions often come with the intense physical signs of transition. It's common to feel some or all of these things:

- overwhelmed, like you can't continue coping with the contractions
- angry and afraid
- grouchy and easily upset
- ready to quit

Luckily, labor is almost over. You need to know that these feelings are normal. You also need to know that you and your baby are all right.

Tanya's Story

Labor was different the second time. It was a lot faster. Also, last time I had pain medicine and couldn't feel anything. This time I felt pain, but I felt like I could handle it. When I got out of the tub, the contractions hurt more. Then my water broke and went all over the floor. I wanted to push right away, but my midwife told me my cervix hadn't opened all the way yet. I couldn't stop pushing. The midwife got me onto my hands and knees, which took away some of the pain and pressure. But I still had to pant a little bit so I wouldn't hold my breath and push. It was really hard. When she told me to go ahead and push, it was such a relief!

Use the same coping methods you used in the active phase (see pages 87–90). It helps to stick with the same rhythmic movements and breathing pattern. This is called a *ritual* (doing the same things over and over). Between contractions, try to relax and rest, if only for a few seconds. There's no need to remain calm and relaxed during contractions. It may be easier if you move and make noise.

Here what your birth partner can do to assist you:

- Stay close to you. (Some women like being held close. Others don't want to be touched at all, but want their partners to be within arm's reach.)
- Keep a rhythm to your breathing. (Your partner can count your breaths, nod in rhythm or have you watch his or her hand while giving you a steady beat.)
- Help you relax between contractions.
- Give you things to help you feel more comfortable (for example, a warm towel on your lower back or belly, a cool washcloth on your forehead, ice chips for thirst, pillows for support).
- Help you feel safe, loved, and protected.
- Call the nurse if you begin to grunt or hold your breath. This may show that you're ready to push.

Jenny's Story

I told the nurse I was feeling pressure in my bottom. Then I got sick and threw up. I got the shakes too. It was really hard. I panicked. The nurse told me to keep my eyes open and look at my mom. The nurse kept saying, "You're okay. This is the hardest part. Keep up with the rhythm." The nurse showed my mom how to count to give me a beat to follow with my breathing and moaning. It was all I could do just to follow my mom. It felt like it would never end, but it did. The next thing I knew I was making grunting sounds and it was time to push my baby out.

Some women really struggle during transition, weeping and crying out for help. Your birth partner may be upset by your pain or the sounds you make and may not know how to help you. Support and advice from your nurse and caregiver can help you both. Your partner may also use the Take Charge Routine. Here's what your partner would do:

- Stay calm. Be confident. (Or at least pretend to be.)
- Hold you or put a hand on your arm to anchor you.
- Not ask any questions, instead giving you gentle suggestions for what to do.
- Encourage you to open your eyes and look at them.
- Say "breathe with me" and give you a rhythm to follow.
- Remind you that labor is almost over and you're doing great.
- Repeat instructions as needed to keep up eye contact and rhythm and to keep you focused on them, not the pain.

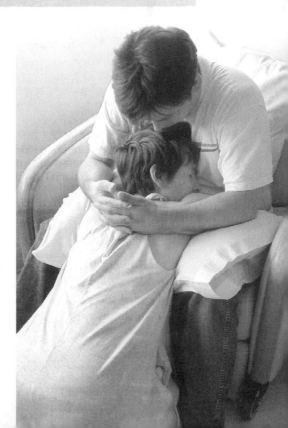

Birth of the Baby: Second Stage of Labor

The second stage of labor (pushing) begins after your cervix has dilated completely. In this stage, your baby moves out of the uterus, down the vagina, and is born. The second stage can be as short as 20 minutes, or it can take more than 3 hours.

In the second stage, you're more like your usual self than you were during transition. You have more energy—sometimes called "a second wind." You're calmer and more relaxed. This is what you can expect your contractions to look like during this stage:

- come every 3–4 minutes
- last about 60 seconds
- be less painful than contractions in transition
- make you feel like pushing (at the beginning of the second stage, you may not feel an urge to push; after 10–20 minutes, when the baby moves down into the vagina, the urge gets stronger)

What Is an Urge to Push?

The *urge to push* feels like a strong desire to grunt and bear down. Many women describe it as feeling as though they have to poop. You can't control the urge, just as you can't control a sneeze. Some women have an urge to push before full dilation. Others don't feel it until the cervix is 10 centimeters. Sometimes a woman never feels it. With an epidural, some women feel a full urge, some feel some pressure, and some just feel "different" from how they felt before.

The pressure of the baby in your vagina causes the urge to push. During each contraction, there are several urges. With each urge, you strain and bear down. Between the urges, you take a few breaths and then push again with the next urge. Between contractions, you won't have an urge to push. So lean back and rest.

When you bear down (push) along with the force of a contraction, it really helps move the baby down. Many women feel better when they push during contractions. Others think it hurts more. If it's painful for you, try another position. Also, try to relax the muscles around your vaginal opening (*perineum*). Pushing works better and is less painful when your birth canal isn't tense.

When the pushing stage begins, some women find themselves holding back. If you're worried about tearing or are uncomfortable having caregivers look at your bottom, ask for warm washcloths to be placed down there—this will help the skin to stretch and cover you up. If you're worried about pooping while pushing, know that it happens often, and your caregivers will wipe it up without even telling you.

Maria's Story

I couldn't believe how hard my body made me push! I pushed for a long time, so my doula and nurse had me try lots of different positions. It was tough. John kept reminding me to relax my bottom. It hurt less when I didn't tighten up.

Positions for Pushing

If you have a short pushing stage, you may only use one position.
But if you push for a few hours, you may try several positions to find
the ones that are comfortable for you and help the baby move down.
When your baby is crowning (the head is visible at your vaginal opening), your doctor or midwife may ask you to get into a specific position
for delivery.

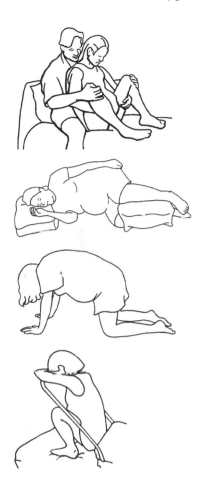

Here are some possible positions. If you do not have pain medications, you are able to use any of them. With pain medications, only
some work.

- Sitting and leaning back is called *semi-sitting*. It's easy for you
  to push in this position even if you have an epidural, and many
  caregivers like it best.
- Lying on your side may reduce back pain. It puts less pressure
  on your rectum or hemorrhoids and means your perineum is less
  likely to tear. Also easy to do with an epidural.
- The *hands-and-knees* position decreases back pain and may
  be the best position for delivering a big baby. If you have an
  epidural, this position is challenging to get into and you'll need
  support, but it's possible.
- Squatting widens your pelvis and helps your baby move down the
  vagina. It can help pushing to go faster. Some hospital beds have
  squat bars to help you get into this position. This position is not
  typically used with an epidural.

Your Baby Is Born

As your baby comes out, the head stretches your vagina open, and you may feel it stinging or burning.
Your caregiver may tell you not to push. To stop pushing, pant or blow out air through your mouth.
Try relaxing your bottom.

The top of your baby's head comes out first, then her face. Once the head is born, it's a relief to have
less pressure and pain. After the shoulders are out, the rest of the baby comes quickly. Your caregiver
may suck fluids out of your baby's nose and mouth with a rubber suction bulb, although this is becoming less common.

After the birth, your baby is
put on your belly and dried off.
The umbilical cord is clamped
and then cut. (It is best to wait a
few minutes after birth to clamp
and cut the cord.) Then you
can hold your baby skin-to-skin
during third stage.

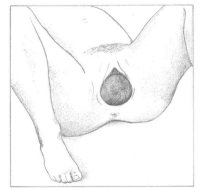

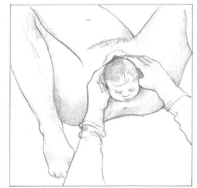

Delivery of the Placenta: Third Stage of Labor

As you get to know your baby, you wait for the placenta to come out. This stage is the shortest and lasts about 10–30 minutes. The contractions aren't usually very painful. You may not notice them because you'll be busy looking at your baby. Or you may have uncomfortable cramping. You may be asked to give a few pushes to get the placenta out. Then, if you've had an episiotomy or tear, your caregiver will stitch it closed. (For more about episiotomies, see page 106.) You are given a shot (of anesthetic medicine) to numb the pain of the stitches.

The First Hours after Birth

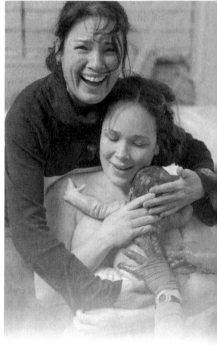

Women have a variety of feelings after the birth. You may feel relieved that labor is over. You may feel proud of how well you did. You may be filled with love for your new baby, or surprised at how he looks. You may be full of energy, or you may just feel tired and want to rest awhile.

Your partner may be overwhelmed with emotion and exhaustion at this time. Your partner and family members may hug you and cuddle your baby. You may all cry with joy. Or you may feel worn out by labor or shocked at the reality of the baby. Sometimes it takes a while for the joy and connection to come.

Focusing on the Baby

Your baby may look bluish at first and be streaked with blood. This is normal. A white, creamy substance (called *vernix*) may cover her body. This protected her skin while she was floating in the bag of waters. Your baby will begin breathing within seconds. Then her skin color will look more normal. Your baby's first cry will make everyone happy!

Right after birth, your nurse or caregiver will check your baby's well-being. This is called an *Apgar* test. If your baby's skin is pink and she's wiggling and crying, she's doing well, and the best place for her to spend her first hour is in skin-to-skin contact with you. Hold your bare baby on your bare chest, with a blanket over both of you. This helps her feel safe and helps get her breathing and her temperature stable. As she nuzzles your chest, it tells your body to release the placenta and start making more breast milk. If the baby is not placed skin-to-skin with you right away, ask for that to happen.

If your caregivers have any concerns about the baby, they'll massage her and possibly give her oxygen. If needed, they may take her to a nearby warming bed for more medical care or to a special care nursery. As soon as possible, they should return her to your chest.

In the first hour after birth, your baby is likely to be calm and alert with her eyes wide open. This is a good time to hold your baby and take a good look at her. She'll notice new sounds, smells, and sights around her.

If you plan to breastfeed your baby, try to begin in the first 30–45 minutes after birth. This is when your baby is alert and interested in feeding. Your nurse can help you.

After feeding, your baby will be weighed and measured. The nurse will check your baby's heartbeat, breathing, and temperature several times after birth. Sometime in the first hour, the nurse will put ointment in your baby's eyes to prevent an infection. Your baby will also get a vitamin K shot to prevent bleeding. If you have any concerns about the ointment or shot, talk to your caregiver before the birth. The nurse will give your baby a bath. This is usually done in the sink in your room. Although many hospitals do the bath in the first few hours, recent research shows that waiting several hours may be better for helping the baby control her temperature and blood sugar. You can ask to wait.

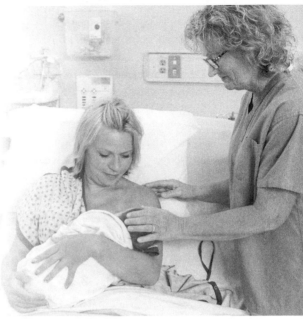

Recovery Time after the Birth

In the first hour or two after the birth, the nurse will check your blood pressure, pulse, and temperature often. After birth, your uterus will continue to contract to close off the blood vessels where the placenta was and to shrink back to its nonpregnant size. The contractions (called *afterpains*) may be uncomfortable enough in the first few days that you'll need to use labor pain techniques or take pain medications, such as ibuprofen. Your nurse or midwife will check your uterus to make sure it remains firm so that you won't lose too much blood. If it is relaxed, she will massage it to make it contract. This can be quite painful. You can ask your nurse to show you how to check it and massage it yourself.

After birth, you'll have a bloody vaginal flow like a heavy period. This is called *lochia*. You'll need to wear a maxi pad. To help reduce pain and swelling in your vagina, the nurse will place an ice pack on your perineum. (See pages 117–118 for more information about afterpains, lochia, and perineal care.)

Soon after the birth, your legs may shake. This is common. A warm blanket will help. The shaking will go away in a short time. You also may feel hungry and thirsty. This isn't surprising—you've been working hard and probably missed some meals. Ask for something to eat and drink.

You'll probably feel relief that labor is over—and excitement that your baby is here.

Note to Fathers and Partners

Supporting your partner through labor may be physically exhausting and emotionally challenging for you. Make sure you take care of yourself as well as your partner. Rest in early labor if she doesn't need your active support, snack to keep your energy up, go to the bathroom when you need to, and ask for support from caregivers, friends, or family. During transition, your partner will really need your full support, so make sure you'll be ready when she needs you most. In the first hour after the birth, the baby will be wide awake and ready to connect. Spend some time with your partner getting to know this new person. There will be plenty of time later to make all the phone calls and e-mail messages announcing the birth.

CHAPTER 7

What about Pain during Labor?

You may be worried about labor pain—most expectant parents are! You may hope to do a natural birth without pain medications. We will talk about the skills you need to help you do that. You may plan on having an epidural for pain relief. We'll give you the information you need when making that choice. You may not know what you want. We'll talk about how to decide.

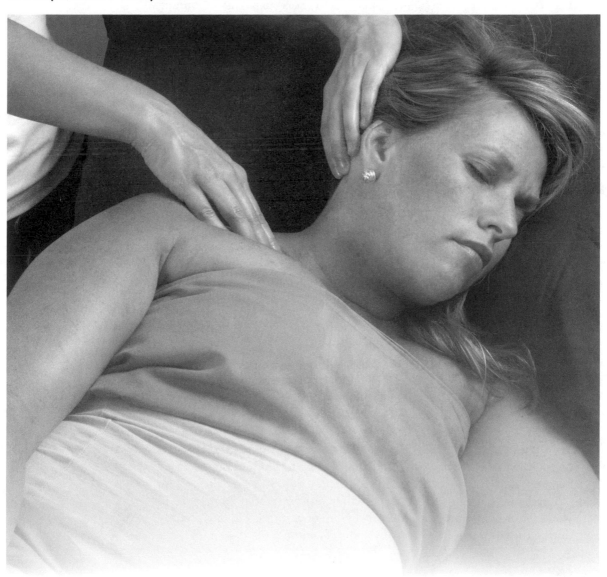

What Causes Labor Pain?

Pain is a normal part of the birth process. Pain during labor does not mean that something is wrong. If you remind yourself of that in labor, you'll probably feel less pain because you're not so afraid. (Fear makes pain worse.) Several things cause childbirth pain:

- Your uterine muscles are working very hard to push the baby down and out. When muscles work hard, they get tired and may burn.
- Your cervix has worked hard for nine months to hold the baby in. Now it is stretching and opening to let your baby out, and that can hurt.
- During birth, your birth canal (vagina) stretches out to let the baby pass through. This is normal, and your body is designed to do it. But the pressure and stretching can be painful.
- Pain is a signal from our bodies about what we need to change in order to be healthy. In labor, pain tells you that you need to get to somewhere safe, and you need to get people to help you. So when you are somewhere you feel safe and you have support, you will have less pain.

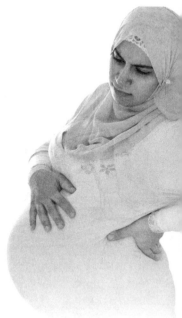

It may help to know that pain isn't continuous in labor. It comes and goes with contractions.

Knowing several pain-coping methods (called *comfort techniques*) helps you feel less afraid. Using these skills during labor helps you feel more powerful. Try practicing the techniques in this chapter during pregnancy so you know how to do them during labor.

Note to Fathers and Partners

Practice comfort techniques together. Make a list of the things that seem to work best for your partner. Also, be sure you know what her goals are for medication. If you know she wants pain medicine as early as possible, you can help her cope through the start of labor and help her get medication once it's available. If you know she doesn't want pain medication, then you'll work hard to support and encourage her when she's in pain.

Follow her lead:

- Look for relaxation. If you do something and she softens and relaxes, then it's helping and you should keep doing it. If she tenses up and turns away, it's not helping. You should stop and try something new on the next contraction.
- Look for rhythm (in her breathing and movement). Whatever she's doing, if she has rhythm, she's coping. If not, you need to help her find a rhythm.
- Support her ritual. Once you have found coping techniques that work for her, keep doing the same thing on each contraction. In labor, there's a lot of uncertainty. It helps her if she can count on you to keep doing what's working for her. When she loses her rhythm or can't relax at any point during the contraction, it's time to find a new ritual.

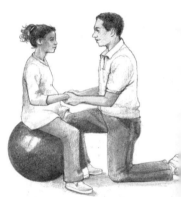

Skills for Coping with Childbirth Pain

There are many ways to cope with the pain and stress of labor. These comfort techniques may be used for your entire labor. Or you can use them to ease your pain in early labor and then use pain medicines if or when they're needed.

There are two different ways we experience pain: *intensity* and *unpleasantness.* Intensity is how much it hurts. Unpleasantness is how much we want to escape from that pain. Some people might also call these parts "pain" and "suffering." When a woman in labor feels safe and supported, and can do the things she needs to do to cope, she may experience pain but not feel as though she's suffering, even if the pain is intense.

Coping well during labor doesn't necessarily mean you don't feel pain. It means that you're not overwhelmed or panicked by the contractions. It means that you're able to relax and handle the pain, even when you can't make it go away. We also call this "working with labor pain."

If you do not use pain medications in your labor, your body will release *endorphins*, hormones that help relieve pain. Your hormones will work best, and labor will hurt the least, if you feel safe and loved, if you don't feel like you're being observed or judged, and if no one disturbs your coping ritual. Learn more about hormones and how they help you work with labor pain by going to http://www.childbirthconnection.org and searching for "Pathways to a Healthy Birth."

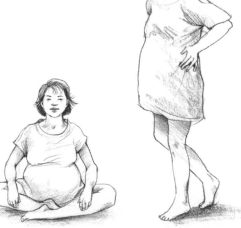

Use Relaxation to Reduce Pain

Women who cope well in labor use *relaxation*. Some women let go of tension and let their muscles go limp during contractions. Then they move around between contractions. Other women are more active during contractions (swaying or rocking) and relax and rest between contractions. Do whatever is relaxing for you at that time of labor.

Here are some ways relaxation can help:
- save your energy (so you don't get so tired)
- calm your mind
- reduce your stress and fear, which reduces pain
- decrease your pain by decreasing muscle tension

The ability to relax comes more easily to some than to others. With practice, however, you can learn to do it. Start by doing the Learning to Relax exercise on page 42. Then try the exercises in this chapter.

When you begin practicing relaxation, do it in a quiet, calm place. Lie down on your side with plenty of pillows or sit in a comfortable chair with your head and arms supported. Try using 1 skill each night before falling asleep. After you've learned to relax in quiet places, practice relaxing while sitting up, standing, or walking. Try relaxing in noisier, active settings. Remember that hospitals are busy places, and labor can be stressful.

Relaxing While You're Resting

You can read this exercise to yourself and think about it as you practice. Or you can have your partner read it to you while you listen.

1. Find a comfortable position. Make sure your head, arms, and legs are supported.

2. Close your eyes and breathe slowly.

3. Think about your toes and feet. Just let go of tension there.

4. Now focus on your legs. They feel comfortable. Think of your legs as warm and relaxed.

5. Focus on your lower back. Imagine that someone with warm hands is giving you a back rub. Feel the warmth. Feel the tension leaving.

6. Pay attention to your chest. As you breathe in, your chest swells easily, making room for the air. As you breathe out, your chest relaxes to help the air flow out. Breathe slowly and let the air flow in and out. This helps you relax more.

7. Focus on your arms. Let go of tension. Relax down your arms to your hands and fingers.

8. Now focus on your neck and shoulders. Your head feels heavy. Feel the tension slipping away.

9. Think about your face. Your jaw is relaxed. Your eyelids are heavy. You have a calm, peaceful expression on your face. This means you're also calm and peaceful inside. Take a few moments to enjoy this calm feeling.

10. Now it's time to end this relaxation session. Gradually open your eyes, wiggle your toes, stretch, and get up slowly.

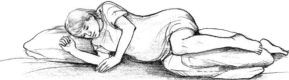

Relaxation Countdown

The relaxation countdown is like a wave of relaxation from your head down to your toes. You can use this countdown to help you get back to sleep at night or whenever you want to quickly release muscle tension during a busy day. During labor, you can use it to *relax* in between contractions.

Sit in a chair or lie down. Close your eyes.

Breathe in through your nose and out through your mouth. As you breathe out, think relax and let go of any tension in your head, neck, and shoulders. Breathe in again. As you breathe out, relax your arm, hands, and fingers. Continue down this list:

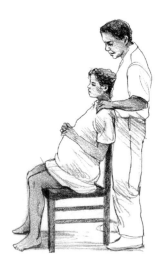

5. Head, neck, shoulders

4. Arms, hands, fingers

3. Chest and belly

2. Back, buttocks, bottom

1. Legs, feet, toes

Then try the rapid relaxation countdown, where you take 1 deep breath in, and on 1 long breath out, you count down from 5 to 1, letting go of all tension in that order.

Notice how you feel. Enjoy the relaxation and the release of tension.

Relaxing Tension Spots

Sometimes it's easier to relax one area of your body than it is to relax your whole body. This technique helps you release tension from the areas you tighten when you're stressed. For example, many people tense their shoulders, clench their jaws, or frown. Relaxing these *tension spots* will reduce your total pain in labor.

- Sit or lie down. Get comfortable.
- Breathe in slowly and easily through your nose. Think about where on your body you are holding tension. Focus there, and when you breathe out through your mouth, release any tension from that spot.
- When that area is relaxed, let your attention go to another area where you feel tense. As you breathe in, notice the tension. As you breathe out, let it go.
- You may notice tension in any of these areas, or elsewhere:
    - eyes and brow
    - mouth and jaw
    - neck and shoulder
    - arms and hands
    - upper back or lower back
    - hips and buttocks
    - legs

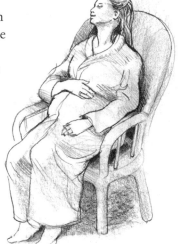

If 1 breath isn't enough to relax an area, take in another breath and release more tension there. Then move on to any other areas where you feel tension.

During a contraction, you may not be able to move through all these areas of your body. Relax as many as you can. You can also ask your partner to rest his or her hand on a tension spot as you breathe in and out or to massage you there. This is called *touch relaxation*.

Women who use coping skills such as relaxation and breathing usually feel less labor pain than women who don't use them. These skills can also be helpful at other times in your life. If you learn them now, you can teach your child to relax and breathe through the pain of a hurt knee or a sore finger. Or you can help yourself or your child through a painful medical procedure such as getting a shot.

Use Rhythmic Breathing to Reduce Pain

During labor contractions, try to breathe in patterns that have a steady beat. Try to combine your special breathing patterns with rhythmic movements (rock, sway, or dance in rhythm) or sounds (moan or chant).

Breathing Patterns for Labor

Breathing patterns have several benefits for labor. They help you relax, help make sure you and your baby get plenty of oxygen, and help you focus on a rhythm. By practicing breathing patterns before labor, it will be easier to use them during labor.

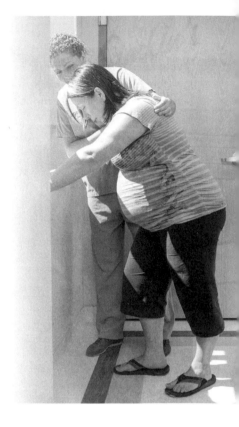

How to Use Breathing Patterns during Labor Contractions
1. When a contraction begins, take a big, relaxing breath.
2. You may choose to keep your eyes open or closed.
3. Relax your muscles as much as you can. With every out-breath, try relaxing more.
4. Breathe in a rhythmic pattern through the contraction.
5. Focus on a comfort measure:
– Look at something.
– Talk silently to yourself, such as counting your breaths.
– Move in rhythm.
– Ask your partner for a massage. Focus on that touch.
– Enjoy the warmth of a shower or bath.
6. At the end of the contraction, take a relaxing breath. Release all your tension as you breathe out.

Slow Breathing

If you don't feel like you need to do anything special to handle the pain of contractions, just breathe normally.

Begin using slow breathing when it's hard to walk or talk during a contraction, and you need to cope with the pain. Use this pattern as long as you can. You may use it through your entire labor, or you may switch to light breathing when contractions get harder to manage.

How to Use Slow Breathing in Labor

1. Slowly breathe in through your nose. Then slowly breathe out through your mouth.
2. Breathe in quietly. Your out-breath should sound like a relaxing sigh.
3. Keep your shoulders relaxed and comfortable.
4. Have your mouth slightly open and relaxed.
5. Breathe about 6–10 times per minute (about half your normal breathing rate).

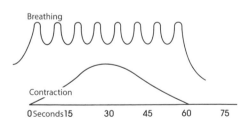

The most important thing is that the slow breathing is comfortable and relaxing for you. Practice this pattern until you can do it easily. Try to do slow breathing for 60–90 seconds, because in labor the contractions last about that long.

Light Breathing

Light breathing is used when you have trouble relaxing or keeping a rhythm using slow breathing.

How to Use Light Breathing in Labor

1. Breathe in and out through your mouth.
2. Keep your breathing shallow, quick, and light. Think about using only the top part of your lungs.
3. When you breathe out, make a short blow with a light sound, such as "hoo" or "hee." Use the sound you like best.
4. Focus on the out-breaths. Let your body take care of the in-breaths. They should be quiet. But you should hear the out-breaths.
5. Take a breath every 1 or 2 seconds.
6. Make each breath about the same. Keep the same rhythm.

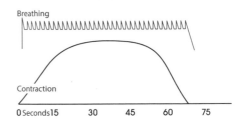

When you first try this, you may feel tense, as if you can't get enough air. Slow your breathing down a bit. Practice light breathing for 1–2 minutes at a time until you can do it without feeling short of breath. Some women say that it is easier to do in labor than in practice sessions.

Light breathing may make your mouth dry. To keep from feeling thirsty, try these suggestions:
- Between contractions, sip water or suck on ice chips.
- During contractions, touch the tip of your tongue to the roof of your mouth.
- After several contractions, brush your teeth, rinse your mouth, or use lip balm.

Other Breathing Patterns

Some women combine slow and light breathing to make new patterns.
1. One way is to take 3 light breaths and then a long, slow one. It would look like this:

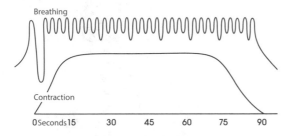

2. Another way is to start with slow breathing and change to light breathing at the peak of a contraction when it's most painful. It might look like this:

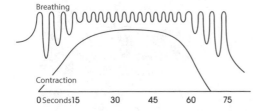

How to Practice Breathing Patterns

During the last months of your pregnancy, try to practice each breathing pattern 2–3 times a week. Try them in a variety of positions. Try mixing them with comfort techniques such as attention-focusing or movement (see pages 86–90).

By practicing, you'll be prepared to use breathing patterns during labor. You may or may not use all of them, but learning them gives you more options for coping with labor pain.

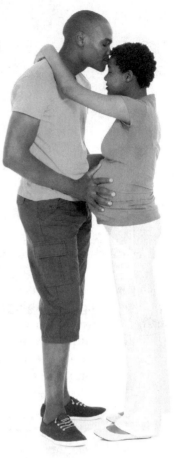

Tanya's Story

When the pain got pretty bad, Jason sat close by, keeping eye contact with me and nodding his head up and down and making me breathe with him. I didn't think I could keep going, but I guess I moved along really well. I didn't even have a chance to wish I could get drugs for pain. When I got to push, all I wanted to do was get the baby out. And I did! I can't believe I did it at home without drugs. I'm proud of myself. My little boy was wide awake, and he looked right at me when he heard my voice. Jason and I spent his first hour snuggling in bed with him. He'll usually have to share us with Molly, so this was our chance to give him our full attention.

Using Positions and Movement to Reduce Pain

Moving around during labor helps in several ways: *doing something* gives you something to think about other than pain, changing positions helps relax sore muscles, and some positions can help speed up a slow labor. Plan to change positions at least every 30 minutes. Use the Road Map on pages 196–197 to remind you of these positions.

- **Resting positions**. Leaning forward will help relieve back pain, and help your baby rotate into the best position (this may speed up labor).
  - lying on your side, or tilted toward your belly
  - leaning over the back of a chair, or the head of the bed
  - hands and knees, or leaning over a birth ball (like those used in exercise classes)

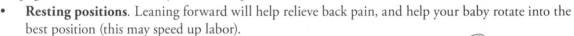

- **Upright and active positions**. These may speed up labor, because they help your baby descend.
  - sitting or standing
  - sitting on a birth ball
  - rocking in a chair or on a birth ball
  - swaying from side to side or slow dancing

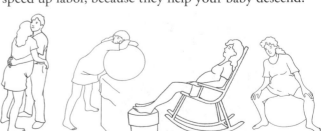

Use Comfort Techniques and Support

In this book, you will learn several comfort techniques that will help you in labor. But you also have an array of coping techniques you already know and use to help you with discomfort. Think about these questions:

- What helps you relax now? (Is it a massage, a bath, a shower, or thinking about pleasant places and activities?)
- What helps you feel safe and comfortable? (Is it a soothing voice or your favorite pillow, music, or photo?)
- What helps you feel better when you're sick or in pain?
- What calms you down when you're worried or scared?

These things will also help you in labor.

Having a Birth Partner

You'll feel more secure if you have a familiar person with you during labor. Also, contractions may seem less painful. During your pregnancy, choose the person you'd like as your birth partner. Some women have more than one. Your birth partner may be the baby's father, your mother, a relative, a friend, or a doula.

What Does a Birth Partner Do?

These are ways your birth partner can help you before the birth:

- go to childbirth classes with you
- listen to you when you talk about your needs and plans for the birth
- help you write a birth plan

These are ways your birth partner can help you during labor:

- help you pass the time during early labor (walking, listening to music, talking, making snacks, and so on)
- drive you to the hospital or birth center
- time contractions
- help you relax between contractions
- help you cope as needed during contractions
  - keep a rhythm for your breathing
  - help you use different positions and movement
  - help you focus your attention away from the pain
- provide or suggesting comfort techniques
  - give you a back rub
  - offer sips of water or ice chips
  - help you get into a tub or shower

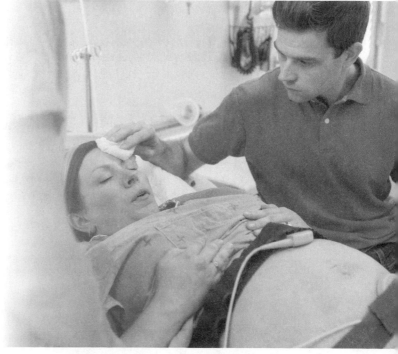

- stay calm and reassuring, offer encouragement
- help you feel safe and loved
- help you ask questions and make informed choices
- share in the joy of birth

If you're going to have more than 1 birth partner, decide what each person's role will be. The one who attended prenatal classes with you may be best at helping you with relaxation and breathing patterns. A family member may be best at offering love and support. A doula may be best at suggesting coping skills and calming both you and your partner. Write down everyone's role in your birth plan.

Maria's Story

Katie, our doula, helped us so much during labor. She reminded me to move around to keep labor going. Then, just at the right time, she suggested that I rest for a while. She seemed to know exactly what I needed. Because I was having a lot of back pain, I also spent a lot of time on all fours swaying my hips. Katie showed John how to press on my back during a contraction. While John was doing that, Katie helped me with my breathing. It was really great to have them both helping me.

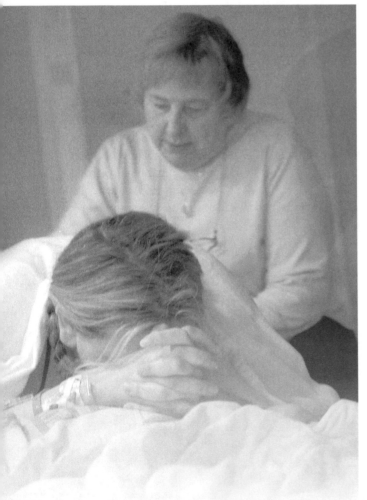

What Is a Doula?

A *doula* is a woman who's trained to help you and your partner by giving support and easing your pain and worries during childbirth. Most professional doulas charge a fee for their services. Many of them have a sliding scale for lower-income families.

The doula's role is to help you have the most satisfying birth possible. She stays with you from the time you call her until 1–2 hours after the birth. She helps you in the ways you want to be helped. She may be your only birth partner, or she may help your loved one or friend to comfort you.

Two great resources for learning more about doulas and finding one in your area are www.dona.org and www.doulamatch.net.

Focusing Your Attention

During labor contractions, you'll want to focus your attention on something. Some women find it helpful to "tune in to" the pain. They focus on it and change their activities to respond to it. Other women "tune out" and think of something other than the pain. To help get your mind off the pain, try focusing on what you notice with your 5 senses:

- *Sight.* Look at something, such as your partner's face, a picture, or a toy for the baby.
- *Sound.* Listen to your favorite music, a soothing voice, or the rhythmic pattern of your breathing.
- *Touch.* Pay attention as your partner touches or strokes you during a contraction. Hold something in your hands, such as a stuffed animal that you can squeeze.
- *Taste.* In early labor, eat a variety of foods. If your hospital only allows clear fluids, try juice, frozen juice bars, Jell-O, or soup broth.
- *Smell.* Bring something that smells good to you (your favorite lotion or a soothing massage oil).

You can also get your mind off the pain by focusing your thoughts on other things:
- Think about the words of a song, poem, or prayer. Or say or sing them out loud.
- Picture yourself in a calm and pleasant place (for example, lying on the beach, walking in the park, or sitting in a cozy chair).
- Count your breaths during each contraction (or have your partner do it). This helps you know when you're near the end of a contraction.

Katie's Story

As a doula, I've sometimes seen laboring people do exactly what they'd planned to do for coping techniques. But often, we end up inventing a spontaneous ritual during labor. One mom made up her own breathing technique, saying "hmmmm—HAAA" through labor. It was a great rhythm, so her husband and I hmm-haaaed right along with her. One mom had a blood draw and ended up holding onto a cotton ball. For the rest of labor, as long as she had her cotton ball, she was relaxed. But if she dropped it, she was really distressed. So one of my big jobs was to keep track of the cotton ball. I don't need to understand why something works; I just trust that it's working. One mom was an engineer, and during labor, she was so busy thinking it was slowing down her labor. So I talked and talked—my babble calmed down her brain enough that she could listen to her body. I could tell that what I was doing was working, because if I was talking, she was relaxed. If I stopped talking, she would tense up.

Use a Counter-Irritant

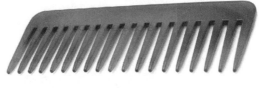

Have you ever noticed yourself coping with one pain by doing something else that hurts a little? For example, biting your lip to distract yourself from the pain of getting a shot? Or pounding a fist into your thigh to take your attention off the pain of a stubbed toe? This is called a *counter-irritant,* because you're focusing your attention on the irritating thing you control (biting your lip) instead of on the irritating thing you can't control (getting a shot). This can make it easier to cope with the pain you can't control. Also, having more discomfort tells your body to release more *endorphins,* hormones that relieve pain.

This works in labor too. In some cultures, laboring people use hairbrushes or combs with wide teeth that they hold and press into their palms. Some people dig their fingernails into their palms; some pull on their hair. If your partner notices you doing this, he or she can help make sure you don't harm yourself, for example, giving you a washcloth to squeeze.

Using Massage and Touch

Having a massage can be soothing and relaxing during pregnancy and labor. Remind your partner to match the massage to the rhythm of your breathing. Work with your partner before labor to find out which kind of touch is most helpful to you:

- light, tickly touch
- *effleurage*—lightly stroking your belly in circles
- firm stroking on your arms, legs, or back
- squeezing and letting go of muscles, such as those in your shoulders or upper arms
- firm massage of your neck, shoulders, back, feet, or hands

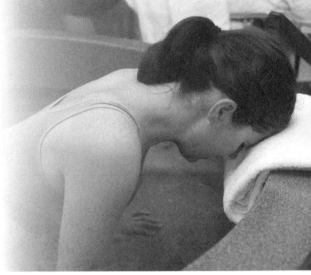

Using Baths and Showers

Being in warm water is very comforting for most women during active labor. Contractions are usually less painful in the water. A shower or whirlpool bath may help you relax by providing a gentle massage.

Using Warm and Cold Packs

A warm pack on your lower back or belly can be very soothing. A warm pack is simply a washcloth or small towel soaked in very warm water, wrung out, and put wherever you need it. You can also use a heating pad or a hot-water bottle.

A cold pack helps reduce back pain during labor. Examples of cold packs include a rubber glove filled with crushed ice, a bag of frozen peas, or a frozen gel pack like the ones used for sports injuries. Wrap the cold pack with a thin towel to protect your skin.

Drinking Enough Fluids

Most women are thirsty during labor. Between contractions in early labor, try to drink something (water, tea, soup, or juice). In active labor, you may not want to drink as much. So take small sips of water or suck on a frozen juice bar.

If the nurses tell you not to drink anything or if you're vomiting, they'll give you IV fluids (see page 71). Even with IV fluids, you may have a dry mouth. Try sucking on ice chips or a sour lollipop, brushing your teeth, or rinsing with cold water or mouthwash.

Your partner can remind you to go to the bathroom about once every hour. A full bladder may slow your labor progress. It also increases pain.

Practicing Coping Skills

Before labor, practice the breathing patterns and relaxation skills in various positions. When you have pregnancy discomforts, test out some of these coping skills to see which help. Some expectant parents also find it helpful to practice these techniques while doing something uncomfortable. For example, holding an ice cube for one minute while practicing attention-focusing options may help you figure out which ones work best for you.

Ways to Cope with Back Pain and Slow Labor

Some people have severe back pain during labor. The techniques in this section help with back pain. They also help with slow labor, especially if you have *irregular contractions* (without a regular pattern you can predict.) On the Road Map (pages 196–197), these labors are shown as the rocky Detour for Labor Pain.

Sometimes back pain is caused by the baby's position. If the back of the baby's head presses on your lower backbones during contractions, you have more pain. When the baby turns around (rotates), back pain usually goes away.

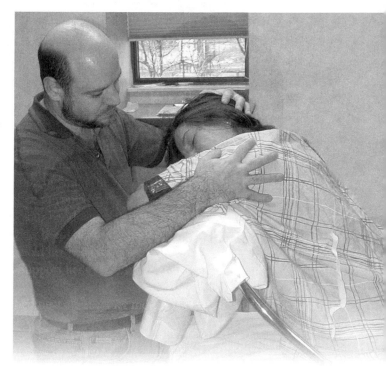

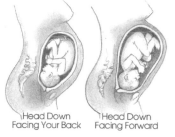

Head Down Facing Your Back   Head Down Facing Forward

Positions to Help Reduce Back Pain

Avoid lying on your back, if possible. These positions can make you feel better:

*   **Being on hands and knees**. Adding rocking movements may help the baby move around to a position that causes less pain.
*   **Leaning forward**. Try leaning forward while sitting, standing, or kneeling. You can lean over a birth ball, the labor bed, or against a chair.
*   **Walking, swaying while standing, and stair climbing**. Movement helps the baby rotate. Being upright also helps the baby move down (descend) into your pelvis.
*   **Side-lying**. Try lying on 1 side and then the other. Find out which side is more comfortable. Roll forward onto pillows.

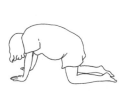
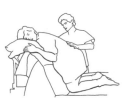
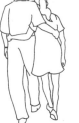
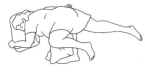

Back Pressure to Reduce Back Pain

Your birth partner can also help by pressing on your back. This external (outside) pressure balances the internal (inside) pressure caused by the baby's head. During a contraction, here's what your partner can do:

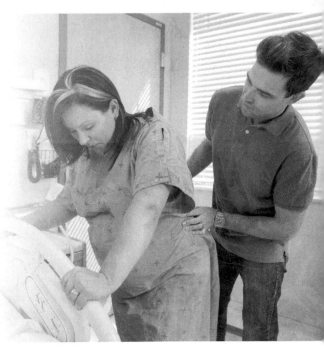

1. Hold the front of one of your hip bones with one hand to keep you from being pushed forward.
2. Press firmly with the heel of his or her hand in 1 spot on your lower back or buttocks. One of the most helpful places to press may be on your sacrum, which is the wide bony area at the bottom of your spine (just above your tailbone).
3. Keep the pressure steady for the whole contraction.
4. Rest between contractions.
5. Ask you how the pressure feels.
6. Stop pressing if the pressure isn't helping or if it hurts you.

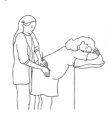

The exact spot that needs pressure may change as the baby moves down into your pelvis. Have your partner press in different spots during a contraction. Tell your partner what feels best.

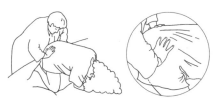

Another type of pressure that may help is the *double hip squeeze*. During a contraction, your partner puts his or her hands on your hips and presses inward.

Maria's Story

I had a lot of back pain during labor, and labor was slow. I used the birth ball quite a bit. I also climbed stairs, and Katie, my doula, showed me how to do something called lunging. When contractions started to really hurt, John pushed on my back, while Katie held my hand. Then my nurse checked my cervix again. I was dilated to 8 centimeters! I stayed on my side for a while and rested. Then it was back to the birth ball and rocking chair. When my baby finally turned around, I didn't like having my back pressed anymore. John was glad because his arms were sore.

Thinking about Pain Medication

During pregnancy, think about whether you want pain medications in labor. Which of these statements best describes your feelings?

- I really don't want pain medications and would be disappointed if I used them. I will need lots of support from my partner with coping techniques.
- I would rather not use pain medication. When labor gets hard, I want my partner to encourage me to continue trying different coping techniques.
- I would like to use coping techniques for as long as possible. When labor gets hard, I will ask for pain medication.
- I would like to have pain medication as early in labor as possible. I need my partner to help me with coping techniques until we reach that point. I want caregivers to offer medication when I can have it.

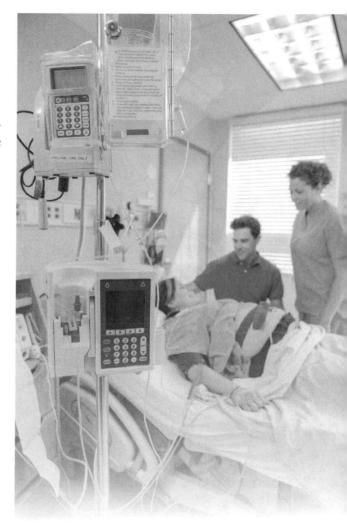

Before labor begins, discuss what you want with your partner and caregiver and put it in your birth plan. But be flexible with your plan. Sometimes what you need in labor may be different than what you expected to need.

The feeling of labor pain is different for each woman. Several things affect how much pain you feel:

- your past experience with pain
- how healthy you are
- hunger, thirst, and whether you're hot or cold
- how long your labor lasts and how tired you feel
- whether you have a birth partner or not
- whether your caregivers are gentle and respectful or not
- your ability to use coping skills to handle the pain

Even if you plan to use pain medication, it's a good idea to learn coping skills. These skills can help you at home in early labor and while you wait to get your pain medicine at the hospital. They also help if you are one of the few women for whom pain medications don't work well.

Even if you plan to not use pain medications, you should learn about their benefits and risks. That way you can make an informed decision if your labor is very long and painful and you decide that you need pain medications to manage.

Pain Medicines Used during Childbirth

Plan to talk to your caregiver about pain medicines during one of your visits in late pregnancy. Labor pain medicines relieve your pain, but they also affect your baby and your labor.

The most common types of pain medicines for labor and birth are *narcotics*, an *epidural*, and *local anesthesia*.

Narcotics

These medicines affect how your brain responds to pain signals from your body. They don't take away all the pain intensity, but they reduce the pain you feel or help you care less about it (make it less unpleasant). You may not notice the pain at the beginning or end of a contraction, but you'll still feel it at the peak of a contraction.

How Are Narcotics Given?

Narcotics are given by *injection* (a shot into a muscle, an IV line, or directly into your vein) or mixed with an anesthetic in your epidural medication. The medicine goes into your bloodstream and through your body. These drugs also go to your baby.

How Do Narcotics Help You?

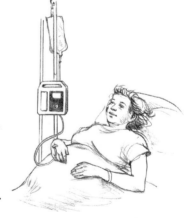

- Narcotics are sometimes used in long prelabor to stop contractions and give you a rest.
- They may be given in active labor to decrease pain and promote relaxation.
- Narcotics are often used for pain relief after a cesarean birth.

What Are the Side Effects of Narcotics?

- They may make you sleepy, dizzy, fuzzy-headed, or sick to your stomach.
- Narcotics can slow labor if given in early labor.
- If given too close to the time of birth, they may affect your baby for the first few hours after birth. Your baby may be sleepier, breathe slower, or need more help with breastfeeding than a baby whose mother did not take narcotics.

Nitrous Oxide

This is a medication you breathe in, also called "laughing gas" which can help you relax and feel less anxious about the pain. It is not widely available, but to learn more about it, see http://www.pcnguide.com.

Epidural

Epidural anesthesia can numb your body from your chest down to your toes or just from your waist to your hips. Epidurals usually take away almost all the pain (reduce the intensity). You may not even notice that you're having contractions. Or you might feel like you're having mild contractions similar to those in early labor.

How Is an Epidural Given?

Drugs are given through a tube that's placed near your *spine* in your lower back.

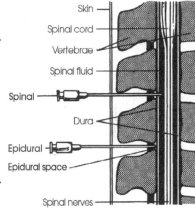

1. You lie on your side with your body curled, or you sit up leaning forward.
2. The doctor (an *anesthesiologist*) washes your lower back and numbs your skin with a shot of *local anesthetic.*
3. A needle is inserted near your backbone in the epidural space. A thin plastic tube is then inserted through the needle. The needle is removed, but the tube remains in place, taped to your back.
4. The tube is connected to a machine that slowly drips the medicines in.
5. Within a few minutes, you begin to notice the effects (tingling, numbness). Within 15–20 minutes, the pain will probably be almost gone.

How Does an Epidural Help You?

- An epidural gives you good pain relief by numbing your belly and back. Very little medicine goes to your baby.
- Epidurals work well for 90–95% of the women who use them.
- It allows you to sleep if you're tired and to think clearly.
- If medical interventions are needed, epidurals can provide pain relief for those. For example, if the need for a cesarean arises, the medication in your epidural can be increased to provide pain relief for the surgery.

What Are the Side Effects of Epidurals?

- An epidural may slow labor progress. You may be more likely to receive Pitocin to speed labor.
- An epidural may cause a drop in your blood pressure.
- You may get a fever, especially if you've had an epidural longer than 6 hours.
- You will probably not be allowed out of bed and will only be able to move in bed with help from others.
- It may be harder to push your baby out.
- The effects of an epidural on you may cause your baby's heart rate to speed up or slow down. This does not harm your baby, but may concern caregivers and lead to more interventions.

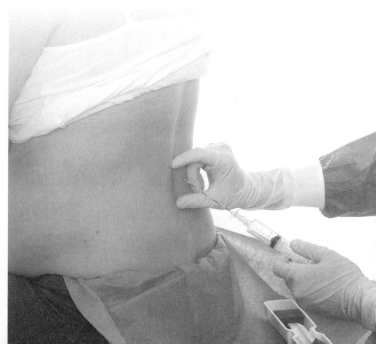

Because epidurals have several side effects, medical procedures are used to keep you and your baby safe. This is what you should expect when you have an epidural:

- Beforehand, IV fluids are given to reduce the chance of a drop in blood pressure. An IV also allows other drugs to be given easily, if needed.
- Your blood pressure and pulse are checked frequently. If your blood pressure drops, you'll receive a medicine in your IV fluids to raise it. You may get an oxygen mask too.
- You'll have an electronic monitor on your belly until your baby is born. This will check your labor contractions and your baby's heart rate.
- A clip will be put on your finger to check your blood oxygen levels. If they're low, you'll be given an oxygen mask.
- A *catheter* (small tube) will likely be put into your bladder to help drain your pee.
- If contractions slow down, your nurse may give you medicine (Pitocin) to increase them.

Labor Support with an Epidural

Although epidurals take away most of the pain, you'll still need support from your partner. You may feel worried and need emotional support. Even if you fall asleep, it's still important for your partner to stay nearby so anytime you wake up, you know you're not alone. If you have side effects, such as itching, nausea, or feeling too hot or too cold, your partner can help with those. They can also help you change positions, which helps labor progress. Try the "epidural roll-over." Spend 20 minutes lying on your left side, then get up onto your hands and knees for 20 minutes, and then 20 minutes lying on your right side. When you're lying on your side, put a pillow or a peanut ball between your legs.

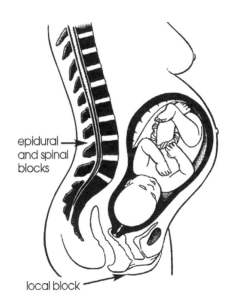

epidural and spinal blocks

local block

Local Anesthesia

Local anesthetics are given as a shot used to numb the area around your vagina. Almost none of the medicine goes to your baby. They are typically not used for labor pain but rather just before birth for an episiotomy or after the birth for stitching.

Cami's Story

After the medications to soften my cervix, the nurse gave me Pitocin to get my contractions going. Labor was really hard. The contractions were long and very painful. And they came so close together. When I reached 6 centimeters, I was exhausted. So I decided to get an epidural. I felt better immediately after that. I didn't have any more pain, so being stuck in bed with an IV wasn't so bad. Pushing was still hard work, but it felt good to being doing something.

Ways to Reduce the Amount of Pain Medicine Used

If you don't want to use a lot of pain medicine, here are some things you can do:

- Take childbirth classes. Practice labor-coping skills so you can use them easily.
- Have a birth partner or doula (or both) help you with labor-coping skills.
- Write your wishes about pain medication in your birth plan.
- When you go to the hospital, ask for a nurse who is expert at caring for women having natural childbirth.
- Make sure you and your partner know how to tell if you're coping well with labor. Can you *relax* between contractions? Can you keep a *rhythm* with your breathing or movement for a whole contraction? Do you have a good *ritual* that's helping you through? If so, you're coping well.

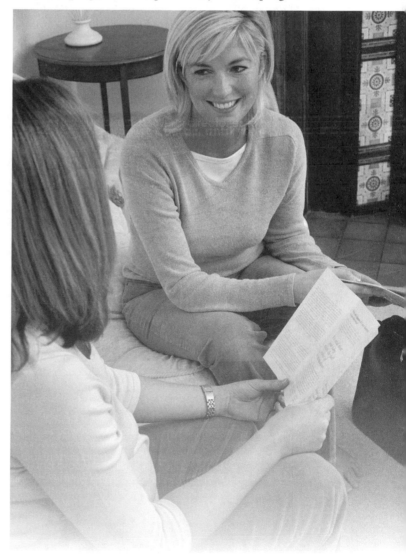

- If you're not coping well, your partner can tell because your muscles will be tight (tense), you won't have a rhythm, and you may sound scared or overwhelmed. Your partner can encourage you to try something new (new breathing pattern, a walk, a bath). Try it for at least 5 contractions, because it takes time for your endorphins (pain-relieving hormones) to kick in.
- When you start thinking about having pain medicine, ask these questions: How far dilated am I? Is labor likely to last much longer? The answers may help you with your decision.
- If you decide to have medicine, ask for a low dose of the drug at first. Use more only if needed.

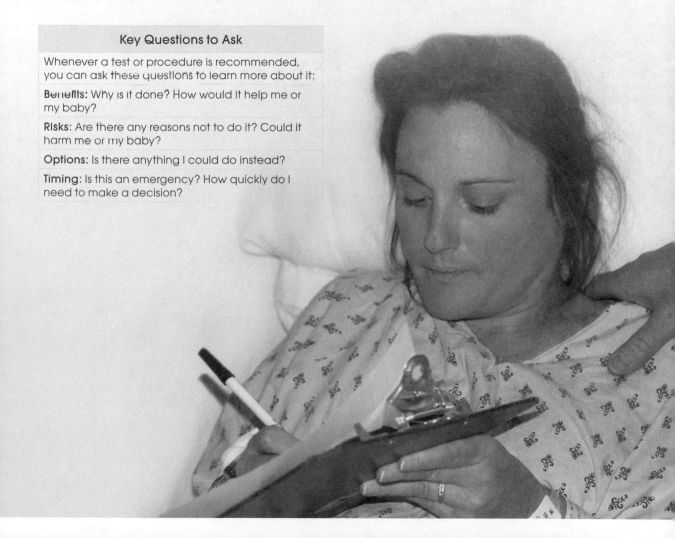

CHAPTER 8

Challenging Labors and Cesarean Birth

You can't know beforehand what your labor will be like. If it goes slower than expected, you may get very tired and discouraged. If it's faster than expected, labor contractions may be hard to handle. This chapter describes different types of labors and births, including cesarean birth. It discusses self-help options you can use to keep labor and birth as normal as possible and to make challenging births easier. It also covers medical treatments that might be recommended. Remember to ask the Key Questions about benefits and risks.

Key Questions to Ask

Whenever a test or procedure is recommended, you can ask these questions to learn more about it:

Benefits: Why is it done? How would it help me or my baby?

Risks: Are there any reasons not to do it? Could it harm me or my baby?

Options: Is there anything I could do instead?

Timing: Is this an emergency? How quickly do I need to make a decision?

Starting Labor

Using medical methods to start labor is called *inducing labor* or *induction*. It might be done if you're overdue, if your water broke but contractions have not begun, or if you or your baby has a health problem that is worsening. If an induction is suggested, make sure you know why.

There should be a medical reason for inducing labor, such as protecting your health or keeping your baby safe. It isn't a good idea to start labor just because it would be more convenient or because you're tired of being pregnant. In that case, induction might cause more harm than good, especially if done before 39 weeks of pregnancy. Learn more about induction at http://www.marchofdimes.org/pregnancy/inducing-labor.aspx.

Jenny's Story

I was at work when my contractions began. They got someone to replace me and someone else to take me to the hospital. But they sent me home. The nurse said my contractions weren't strong enough and were too far apart. I just hung out at my mom's place. We went for walks and watched some TV. That night, even though the contractions were 8 minutes apart, I was in major pain. Kyle took me in to the hospital. They said it was "false labor." There was nothing false about those contractions. They gave me a sleeping pill. The pill did help me get a little sleep. My friend came over and sat with me and helped me cope. On Wednesday, I went back to the hospital. I was finally in true labor, and I got to stay.

What You Can Do When Labor Is Slow to Start

If you've gone past your due date, you may want to try the following methods to start labor. They may not work as quickly as medical methods, but they typically have fewer side effects.

Brisk walking may help start true labor when you're having prelabor contractions. However, walking is better at keeping labor going than starting it. Walk if you enjoy it, but don't tire yourself out.

Sex causes contractions of the uterus, especially when you have an orgasm. Also, semen has a substance in it called *prostaglandin*, which is the same thing your body makes to soften your cervix. If you're not ready for labor, this will not start labor. But when you're close to your due date, sex may help to get labor started. If you choose to have sex, focus on enjoying yourself, not on starting labor.

If your bag of waters has broken, don't put anything into your vagina (including your partner's penis or fingers). (It's okay to do other things that bring you to orgasm.)

Rubbing your nipples makes you produce more *oxytocin* (the hormone that causes your uterus to contract). This method, called *nipple stimulation*, may help to start labor. You can lightly stroke or rub a nipple with your fingertips or a soft washcloth. Or you can roll one or both nipples between your fingers. Within a few minutes, you may feel uterine contractions. Stop if contractions become painful, last longer than 1 minute, or come every 5 minutes or less. Tell your caregiver if you plan to do this because it

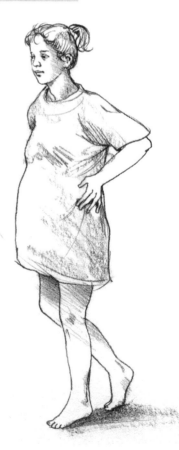

sometimes causes contractions that last too long or come too close together. You can do this several times a day for a few minutes each time.

Acupuncture or acupressure, a traditional Chinese medicine used by a trained provider, can help to start labor with few side effects.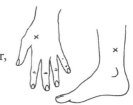

Herbs, homeopathic remedies, and castor oil can be used to start labor; however, only use these with the support of a trained professional (such as a midwife or naturopathic doctor). You should not trust advice you find on the Internet about these remedies.

Medical Methods to Start Labor

There are several methods doctors and midwives use to induce labor. Here are the most common ones:

Prostaglandin can help ripen (soften) the cervix. The drug is similar to the prostaglandin hormone made by your body. It comes in different forms—as a gel, a tampon-like device, or a pill that is inserted into your vagina, or as a pill that you swallow. Prostaglandin is often used before Pitocin is started to make the cervix more ready to open with the contractions. A nurse watches you closely for 2 hours after this method is used.

Pitocin (a drug that's like the oxytocin made by your body) is given to cause the uterus to contract. Pitocin is given by an IV drip at the hospital. The nurse usually starts at a low dose and steadily increases it. The goal is to have contractions that are similar to those in active labor.

Starting labor with Pitocin can be more stressful than allowing labor to start normally. It may take several hours before contractions start. But when they do, they may be close together and painful. These contractions can be hard to handle and emotionally draining.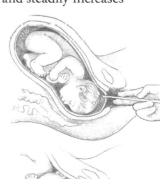

Artificial rupture of the membranes (AROM) means breaking the bag of waters with a plastic *amnihook*. This method is not typically used to start labor, but it's used during labor to speed up labor progress.

A *Foley catheter* or a *balloon catheter* can be inserted into your cervix, then inflated. The aim is to stretch your cervix open. When it begins to open, the catheter falls out, which may start labor.

Cami's Story

My blood pressure kept getting higher, and my doctor wanted to start labor. It wasn't what I had hoped for, so I asked a lot of questions. In the end, I decided it was the best answer for me and my baby.

Induction took a long time, though. First, they used the gel because my cervix wasn't ready to open.

Then I waited. Chris and I played cards and watched TV. Later they gave me Pitocin in an IV. Contractions got a lot harder. I yelled, "Turn off the TV now!" I didn't want any noise. Later they broke my bag of waters. It was all I could do to deal with the strong pains. The contractions came one after another, and I had trouble coping with them. I was lucky that my blood pressure was okay through all that.

Short, Fast Labor

Though a short labor may sound good, it's often overwhelming. When labor lasts less than 3 hours, the early phase has usually passed unnoticed. Then you find yourself in active, hard labor and feel unprepared for the painful contractions. Your partner may be surprised at your reaction to what is supposed to be early labor. Do your best to tell your partner and your nurse how they can help you. (*Note:* These fast labors are fairly rare. The average labor for a first-time mom is 14 hours long.)

What You Can Do If You're in Very Hard Labor

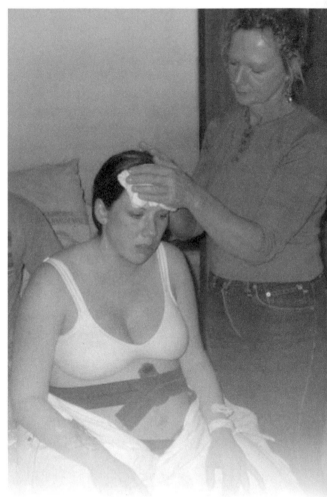

- Don't give up on yourself. Trust your ability to get through this.
- If you begin labor with contractions less than 4 minutes apart and more than 1 minute long, and already strong enough that it's hard for you to cope, quickly go to the hospital or birth center.
- Try not to tense up with painful contractions. Instead, try to relax as much as possible. Use light breathing.
- You'll need help from your partner, nurse, or doula in handling the painful contractions. It may be difficult to use comfort techniques in this intense labor.
- Have a vaginal exam before you make any decision about pain medicines. If you're very close to having your baby, you may decide not to have any medicine.
- You may have the urge to push before your caregiver is ready. If this happens, lie on your side rather than using an upright position and pant. Or only bear down gently.
- After the birth, you'll probably feel relieved but stunned that labor is over so quickly. If you can't remember much about your birth, talk to your partner or caregivers. They can share their memories with you.

What If Your Baby Is Coming Before You Can Get to the Hospital?

Sometimes labor is so fast that you can't get to the hospital in time. Or your midwife arrives late for a home birth. When this happens, babies are born without medical care. Luckily, this doesn't happen often. And when it does, it almost always turns out okay.

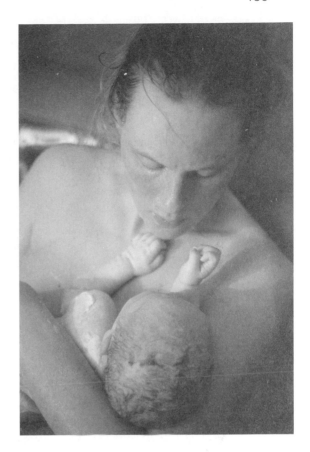

If labor is going very fast, try to get to your birthplace. However, if you feel your body pushing and you can't stop it, or if you can see or feel the baby at the vaginal opening, then you need to stay where you are. If you're home, stay home. If you're in a car, pull to the side of the road. Then follow these steps:

1. Call 911. Get help, if possible. Call your partner or someone nearby.
2. Wash your hands, if possible. Gather clean sheets, towels, or extra clothing. Put something under your bare bottom.
3. Lie down on your side or sit leaning back. Make sure you have enough room for your baby to lie down when she slips out of the birth canal.
4. Pant through each contraction until your baby is born. Try not to hold your breath.
5. After your baby comes out, take these actions:
   - Wipe away the mucus from her nose and mouth.
   - Place her on your bare chest or belly.
   - Keep her warm using a blanket, towel, or piece of clothing.
6. Do not cut the cord. Let your baby nuzzle or suckle on your breast.
7. After the placenta comes out, place it near your baby (still attached by the cord) in a bowl, newspaper, or cloth.
8. Place towels or a pad between your legs to soak up the blood flow.
9. Get medical help as soon as possible to check both you and your baby.
   - If you're in the car, continue onto the hospital.
   - If you're at home, call the hospital to let them know you're coming. Wait until the placenta is delivered before going.
   - If you had planned a home birth, call your midwife so she can come and check on you and your baby.

Long, Slow Labor

Long, drawn-out labors are more common than fast ones, especially if this is your first baby. If you have a long labor, you may become discouraged and very tired.

Long Early Labor

A long prelabor or early phase (1–5 centimeters dilation) is not usually caused by a medical problem. And it doesn't mean that the rest of your labor will be extra long. In most cases, labor progresses normally once you reach the active phase.

What You Can Do for a Long Early Labor

Here are tips for how to handle a slow to start labor:

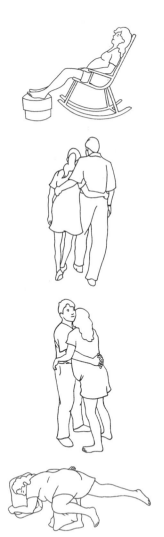

- Don't focus too much on labor. Time 4 or 5 contractions in a row (see pages 65–66). Then wait a few hours (or until your labor pattern changes) before timing again.
- Think of something to help keep your mind off the contractions. Try taking a walk, watching a movie, going shopping, or cooking.
- Try not to become discouraged or depressed.
- Eat and drink. Also, try to rest. You probably won't be able to sleep. If you are very tired, a warm bath may slow you r contractions and let you get more rest.
- Once you've rested, try being more active again. Try methods to help speed up your labor, such as walking, having sex, or nipple rubbing (see pages 100–101). Try not to get too tired. After an hour of activity, sit down to rest.
- Have kind, supportive people around you to help you feel safe and loved. Emotional stress (anger, worry, tension) slows labor progress. Try using relaxation techniques and slow breathing to feel calmer and ease the pain.
- If you have a vaginal exam, ask questions. Find out if your cervix is soft. Ask how much your cervix has thinned. Remember that your cervix needs to be soft and thin before it begins to open.

Medical Care during a Long Early Labor

If your contractions tire you out or if it takes more than 24 hours to get to 3 centimeters dilation, your caregiver may suggest drugs, such as a sleeping pill, or a narcotic shot, such as morphine, to try to slow the contractions and give you time to rest.

A slow early labor is not a medical problem and usually does not need medical treatment. Your caregiver could try induction methods to make contractions stronger (see page 101), but it's usually better to wait for labor to speed up on its own.

Long Active Labor

Dilating from 4 to 6 centimeters can be slow, taking as long as 5–7 hours. After 6 centimeters, progress will speed up.

If labor slows down after 6 centimeters and you go for several hours with no change in dilation, your doctor or midwife may suggest medical methods to speed up labor.

What You Can Do to Prevent or Treat a Long Active Labor

The solution will depend on the problem. Here are possible ways to encourage labor progress:

- If you're thirsty, drink. If you have a full bladder, go to the bathroom. Try to pee every hour to give more space for your baby to descend.
- If you've been in bed for 30 minutes or more, try walking, swaying, or standing. (See page 86 for positions that may help.)
- If you need to stay in bed, change positions about every 30 minutes. Try lying on 1 side, sitting up in bed, or getting on your hands and knees.
- If your contractions are weak, try nipple rubbing or walking.
- If you're tense, try a bath, massage, or shower.
- If you're anxious, talk about your fears. Fear increases pain and can slow labor. Sharing your worries can help.

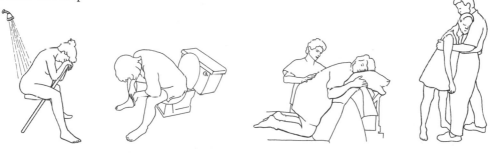

Tanya's Story

At my daughter Molly's birth, labor seemed scary, and that made the pain worse. And my labor was so slow! I think I should've taken a birth class before Molly was born. I would have known more about what was happening. I am less afraid with this baby because I know what to expect.

Medical Care When Active Labor Is Very Slow

During a long active phase, your caregiver will pay close attention to your labor progress.
- You'll probably have vaginal exams to check for cervical dilation and the baby's movement.
- Your baby's health will also be closely watched. Your caregiver will check your baby's heart rate frequently with an electronic fetal monitor. If your baby's heart rate shows problems, your caregiver will try one of the following options to give your baby more oxygen:
  - having you roll over or get on your hands and knees

- – using *amnioinfusion*—putting water back into your uterus to replace the water that came out when your bag of waters broke
- – giving you an oxygen mask
- You may want medicines for relaxation and pain relief if your labor is very long. If you're really tense due to pain, medications can help you relax and that can speed up your labor.
- Your caregiver may break your bag of waters to help speed labor.
- Also, you may be given Pitocin to make your contractions stronger and closer together. If you were planning a home birth, you'd need to go to the hospital for Pitocin.
- If labor does not progress for 6 hours, even with Pitocin, a cesarean birth may be necessary.

Long Second Stage

Although the average pushing stage is about an hour and a half for a first time mom, it's not unusual for pushing to take 3 hours or even more if she has an epidural or if the baby is not in a good position.

You can do these things to try to speed up pushing:

- try a variety of positions (see page 86)
- sit on the toilet for a few minutes to help you remember how to relax your bottom and push at the same time
- rub your nipples to strengthen contractions
- use a mirror to see your pushing efforts or reach down to touch your perineum and baby's head—this can help you see when you're pushing well

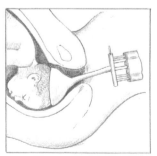

If pushing lasts more than 3 hours with no progress or there are concerns about you or the baby, you may need medical help to get the baby out. Sometimes a caregiver does an episiotomy to make the vaginal opening larger and shorten the pushing time. An *episiotomy* is a cut made with scissors from your vagina toward your rectum. After the birth, this cut is closed with stitches.

Other medical procedures may also be used. A *vacuum extractor* (plastic suction cup) or *forceps* (metal tongs) may be used to help deliver your baby's head. During a contraction, while you push, the doctor pulls with the vacuum or forceps to help your baby come down. These methods are generally safe for you and the baby, but they may cause bruises or sore spots on your baby's head. Also, if forceps are used, you will need an episiotomy.

Talk to your caregiver about these procedures before birth. While most women would prefer not to have these procedures, they are safer than having a cesarean, which is what would happen if they are not used.

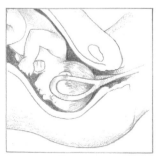

Forceps   Vacuum Extractor

Cesarean Birth

A *cesarean birth* is the surgical delivery of your baby through an incision in your lower belly and uterus. This is also called a *cesarean section* or *C-section*. Because cesarean birth is major surgery, it's usually done only if there's a medical reason. If there's no medical reason for a cesarean, a vaginal birth is safer for both you and your baby.

As you read this section, think about what you would choose if a cesarean became necessary. Then write down your choices in your birth plan.

Reasons for Having a Cesarean Birth

Sometimes the need for a cesarean is known before labor begins. Other times a cesarean is done because of problems that come up during labor.

Reasons Why a Cesarean May Be Planned before Labor Begins

- The mother has *placenta previa* (see page 33).
- The baby is in a *breech position* (see page 62) or *transverse* (lying sideways in the uterus).
- There are triplets or more babies (twins may be able to be born vaginally, depending on their positions).
- The mother has had a cesarean before. If the problem that caused the first cesarean still exists, the mother may need a repeat cesarean. If not, a *vaginal birth after cesarean* (VBAC) is generally a safe option.
- The mother has medical problems that make vaginal birth unsafe. Some examples include heart disease, an active genital herpes infection, or HIV-positive status.
- The baby has a birth defect that would be made worse with a vaginal birth.

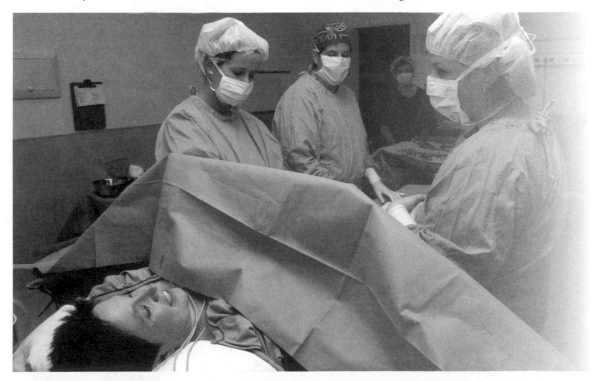

Reasons for an Emergency Cesarean (All Rare)

- placental abruption (see page 33)
- cord prolapse (the umbilical cord is coming through the cervix before the baby, and contractions press the baby onto the cord; this means the baby gets less oxygen)
- other emergencies where the mother or baby are at risk

Reasons an Unplanned Cesarean May Be Recommended during Labor

- Active labor is very slow, and the cervix is opening slowly. Because early labor is usually slow, it's a problem only when labor slows down after 6 centimeters dilation and stays slow for hours. (Sometimes this "failure to progress" can be fixed—see pages 91–92.)
- The second stage is very slow and isn't progressing. This means the baby isn't coming down through the birth canal. This usually doesn't mean the baby is too big. It often occurs because the baby's head is tilted or turned in such a way that it doesn't fit through the pelvis. (Sometimes the mother can fix the problem with the baby's position by changing her own position. Sometimes the caregiver can use his or her hand to turn the baby's head.)
- There are concerns about the baby's heart rate. The baby's heart rate is faster or slower than normal, or is not responding to contractions as expected (also known as *indeterminate* or *abnormal heart rate tracings*). The baby may be doing fine, and there may be no reason to worry, or the changes in the heart rate might show the baby is not getting enough oxygen. If caregivers are concerned about the baby's well-being, they may recommend a cesarean.

Cami's Story

Once the induction worked, labor moved along really well. Then when it was time to push, I was happy. I thought we'd be seeing Tommy soon. Well, I pushed and pushed for I don't know how long. My doctor checked my progress while I pushed—putting her fingers inside me to feel the baby's head. She said the baby was stuck and wasn't coming down. She said that we might need to do a cesarean. Chris knew I hadn't wanted this and asked if there were other things we could try for a little while longer.

I tried using a mirror, and I tried changing positions to see if that would help, and it didn't. Then Tommy's heart rate started to drop. The doctor said, "You've worked so hard and done a good job. But for your baby's sake, we should do a cesarean." I couldn't believe it! How could I be so close and not get my baby out? I cried, and Chris held me and cried too. But I knew they were right. So we decided to do the cesarean.

Side Effects of a Cesarean Birth

When certain problems arise, like those listed on page 108, a cesarean birth is the safest option. This leads some women think it would be quicker and easier to have a cesarean even if there aren't problems. But when you and your baby are healthy, a vaginal birth is the best choice. A cesarean isn't as easy on the mother and baby as you might think. A cesarean is major surgery and carries some possible risks:

- pain for several weeks after the birth
- greater risk of infection and more blood loss than with a vaginal birth
- problems related to the anesthesia used for surgery
- harder time taking care of your baby in the early weeks
- more problems with a future pregnancy (including problems getting pregnant again and having a healthy placenta, and an increased risk of cesarean for the next birth)
- babies born by cesarean have less contact with their mothers in the first hour of life, they're more likely to have breathing problems at birth, and they're more likely to have trouble breastfeeding

If a cesarean is recommended to you, make sure you ask the Key Questions (see page 99). This will help you understand the benefits and risks, and let you learn whether there are any other possible choices to make. If the medical benefits of a cesarean are greater than the medical risks, then it is a smart choice to make, even if it wasn't what you expected.

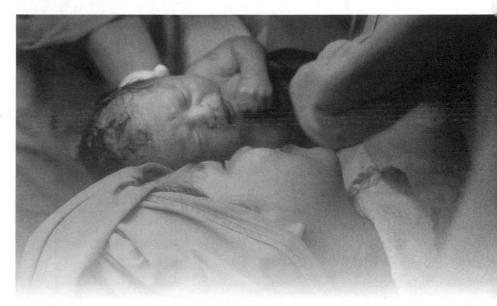

What Happens during a Cesarean?

Before the cesarean birth, your nurse will explain what happens during the operation. You'll be asked to sign a consent form giving your permission for surgery.

The nurse will start an IV in your hand. She'll shave your belly around where the incision will be. You'll be given an antacid to drink. A fetal monitor will be placed on your belly to check on your baby.

Next, you'll be moved to the surgery room. The *anesthesiologist* (a doctor who gives anesthesia) will talk with you about pain medicines. If you already have an epidural, he or she will increase the amount of medicine you are receiving. Otherwise, you may be given a spinal anesthetic, which is a shot into the area near your spinal cord. Either medication will numb you from your lower chest to your feet and allow you to be awake without feeling any pain.

Nausea, shaking or trembling, and a drop in blood pressure often happen with epidural and spinal anesthesia. Make sure to tell your caregivers if you're cold, nauseous, scared, feeling pain, or feeling like you're having trouble breathing. They can help you feel better.

After the anesthetic has made you numb, the nurse will put a small tube (*catheter*) into your bladder to keep it empty. The IV and catheter and epidural catheter are removed within 24 hours after the surgery.

During the surgery, you lie on your back tilted a bit to 1 side. The nurse washes your belly with an antiseptic (a germ-fighting soap). Then a surgical sheet with a hole near your belly is put over your body. Also, a drape is hung between your head and belly. This keeps the surgical area clean and keeps you from seeing the surgery. Your partner stands or sits near your head. He or she can hold your hand, talk to you, and help you use slow breathing to remain calm.

You may be surprised at all the people and equipment needed for a cesarean delivery. Besides you and your partner, there will be 2 doctors who do the surgery, an anesthesiologist, 1 or 2 nurses, and sometimes additional staff to care for your baby. There are several ways to check on your safety during the surgery:

- a blood pressure cuff on your arm
- heart rate monitors on your chest
- a soft clip on your finger to check your oxygen level

Cami's Story

I was scared, but the cesarean wasn't so bad. Chris was with me and held my hand. There were a lot of people there—3 doctors and a bunch of nurses. It was cold in the room, and I had the shakes. The anesthesia doctor talked to me and gave me something to stop my shaking. I could feel some pushing and pulling in my belly, but it didn't hurt.

I couldn't believe how quickly the baby came out! It seemed like they had just started when I heard him cry. Then I cried. I thanked everybody in the room.

During a cesarean, the doctor makes 2 incisions (cuts): 1 through your skin and the other through your uterus. Your abdominal muscles aren't cut; they're spread apart. You won't feel any pain during the surgery. But you may feel some pressure, tugging, and pulling.

The doctor lifts your baby out and suctions mucus and fluid from her nose and mouth. The doctor cuts and clamps the cord and gives you a quick look at your baby. Your baby is then placed on a warm bed. The nurse dries her and makes sure she's doing well.

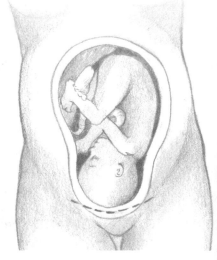

As long as your baby is healthy, your partner can hold her close to you or put her on your chest. You can ask to hold her skin-to-skin. You might be able to breastfeed, with help. If your arms are strapped down, ask about having an arm free to touch her. You can enjoy seeing and touching your baby while the doctor is finishing the operation.

A cesarean takes about 45 minutes. The baby is usually born 5–15 minutes after surgery begins.

After the birth, Pitocin will likely be added to your IV to make your uterus contract to prevent heavy bleeding. When your doctor is removing your placenta, you may feel some pressure or tugging. It takes about 30 minutes for the doctor to close the incisions in your uterus and belly. A thick pressure bandage will be placed over your incision.

The First Hours after a Cesarean Birth (Recovery)

During the first hours after your cesarean, you'll be in your hospital room or a recovery room. The nurse will watch you closely until the anesthesia wears off, checking your blood pressure and well-being often. As long as your baby is doing well, he may stay with you. You'll be able to hold and admire him. You'll also be able to breastfeed. Ask for help getting started.

Cami's Story

After the baby came out, they still had to sew me up. I got the shakes again and felt sick to my stomach. The doctor told me that this was common with cesareans. He said to take a few deep breaths and breathe through my mouth.

At least I could see Tommy. They sucked the mucus out of his nose and mouth and he cried really loud. Then Chris got to hold him. Chris brought him over to me and I said, "Hi, Tommy" and kissed him.

Chris reminded our doctor that we had asked if we could have baby skin-to-skin in the OR and maybe even start breastfeeding. The anesthesiologist said yes. And we did! Holding my beautiful baby made everything okay.

Pain Relief after a Cesarean Birth

The first few days after a cesarean are the most difficult. Pain in your incision will bother you a lot at first, but it will gradually decrease. You may need pain medicine for several days to a week. There are 2 common ways to treat your pain during the first day after surgery:

- Narcotic medicine is put into the epidural catheter. This gives you good pain relief for about 24 hours and doesn't make you sleepy or drowsy. However, itching and nausea are possible side effects. Your nurse can give you other medicine for these, but it might make you sleepy.
- *Patient-controlled analgesia (PCA).* A narcotic goes into the fluid in your IV. Whenever you need pain relief, you press a button to get a small dose of the medicine. The PCA machine is set up to give only the dose ordered by the doctor (and only as often as it's safe). This provides faster pain relief than if you had to ask a nurse for a pain shot. However, IV narcotics may make you sleepy.

After the first day, most mothers use pain pills. At first, they contain narcotics. Later, they contain a medicine such as acetaminophen (Tylenol) or ibuprofen (Motrin). Taking pain pills may make it easier for you to move around, feed, and care for your baby. When the pain is gone, stop using them. Ask your doctor or pharmacist how to dispose of the extra medication.

You might wonder if it's safe to take strong pain medicine while you're breastfeeding. It's fine. Only a small amount goes to your baby through your breast milk.

Recovery from a Cesarean Birth

In the first days after a cesarean, you'll need help doing almost everything. Your incision will hurt, and it'll be hard to move around. Your partner may be able to stay in your hospital room to help with baby care. If a family member can't stay, the nurse will help you as you recover from surgery.

Here are a few ways to be more comfortable during the early days of your recovery:

Rolling over: To make rolling from your back to your side easier and less painful, try this method (called *bridging*):

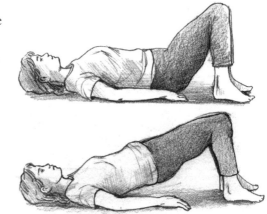

1. Bend your knees 1 leg at a time so your feet are flat on the bed.
2. Lift your hips while keeping your feet and shoulders on the bed.
3. Twist your hips to 1 side while rolling your shoulders to the same side.
4. Now you're lying on your side.

Standing and walking: When you first get out of bed, your nurse will help you. You'll probably feel weak and lightheaded. Try these things to reduce the dizziness:

*   Sit on the edge of the bed and move your feet in circles before standing up.
*   Slowly stand up. Try to stand as straight as you can. It won't harm your incision even though it hurts.
*   Take a short walk after you get used to standing up.
*   Take a slightly longer walk each time you get out of bed.

Going to the bathroom: Sometimes it's difficult to pee after having a catheter in your bladder. If you have trouble, try these things:

*   Pour warm water over your perineum to help start the flow.
*   Pee in the shower or tub.
*   Cough to help start the flow while sitting on the toilet. (If coughing makes your incision hurt, gently press against your incision with your hand to support it while you cough.)

Dealing with gas pains: Having a cesarean can cause gas in your stomach and bowels. If you have gas pains, getting in and out of bed helps. Walking or rocking in a chair helps too. Avoid eating foods that cause gas.

Home after a Cesarean

You'll stay in the hospital 2–4 days. You won't be back to normal by then, however. You'll still be sore, weak, and tired. It takes time to recover from a cesarean birth. Try to have help at home for the first few weeks with meals, baby care, and housework.

After a cesarean birth, you may feel relieved and thankful. Or you may feel sad, disappointed, or angry. If you have trouble adjusting emotionally, talk with your partner or caregiver. You may want to be told again why the cesarean was necessary. Or you may just want to talk honestly and openly about the birth and your feelings. Talking with others may help you overcome your feelings of anger or sadness. You can find support at http://www.ican-online.org.

Planning for Future Births

If you have another baby in the future, you will be able to choose whether to have a repeat cesarean or a vaginal birth after cesarean (VBAC). Several health organizations agree that VBAC is a safe option for most women.

To learn more about cesareans, read "What Every Pregnant Woman Needs to Know about Cesarean" at http://www.childbirthconnection.org/pdfs/cesareanbooklet.pdf.

Note to Fathers and Partners

If labor and birth go very differently than she had hoped, the new mom may need extra emotional support from you to get over the anxiety, guilt, or disappointment. If she has a physically challenging birth or a cesarean, she may need extra physical support from you and other loved ones while she recovers.

Conclusion

Labor and birth happen in many different ways. No one knows ahead of time if childbirth will be fast or slow or have problems. You usually don't know whether your baby will be fine or have a health problem. By learning about the many differences in labors and births, it'll be easier to cope with whatever happens.

CHAPTER 9

Home with
Your New Baby

After the birth, your body goes through some normal physical changes as you recover from pregnancy. You will also experience a lot of emotions as you begin this new phase in your life. This chapter describes what it's like to be a new mother in the first few weeks and months after birth. These early months are called the *postpartum period*.

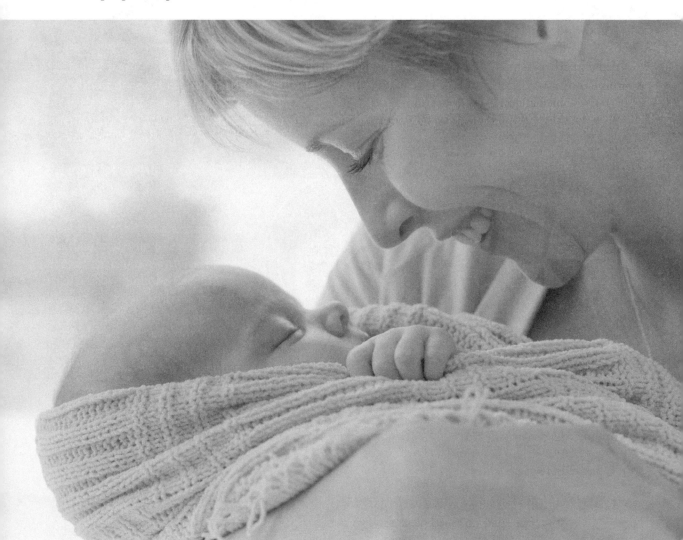

Going Home

Most new mothers leave the hospital about 1 or 2 days after the birth. If you have a cesarean birth, you can expect to stay about 2–4 days. If either you or your baby needs more medical attention, you may stay longer. At an out-of-hospital birth center, you'll go home 1–4 hours after the birth. With a home birth, the midwife leaves 2–4 hours after the birth.

Plan to have comfortable clothes for you and your baby to wear when you go home and a car seat for your baby. (See the packing list on page 57.)

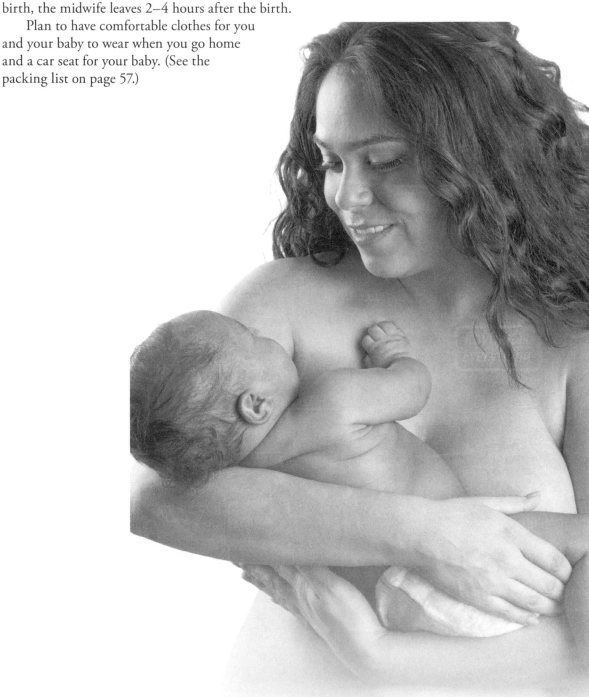

Caring for Yourself

After having your baby, you'll look and feel very different than before you were pregnant. By 6 weeks after birth, you'll probably start feeling "normal" again. It may take a little longer to get back to your old size and shape.

What to Expect in Your Changing Body

These are some of the normal physical changes in the first weeks after the birth.

Your Uterus

When you're not pregnant, your uterus is about the size of a pear. Right after the birth, it's about the size of a large grapefruit. If you touch your belly near your bellybutton, you can feel the top of your uterus. Gradually, your uterus gets smaller. After 6 weeks, it's almost back to its usual size.

In the first days after birth, you'll have *afterpains*. These contractions, which feel like strong menstrual cramps, keep the uterus firm and tight. This helps stop bleeding from the area where the placenta used to be. If it were to relax and feel softer, you would bleed more. Your nurse or midwife may massage your uterus to make it contract; breastfeeding also causes more contractions. If you've had a baby before, these cramps may be more painful this time around. To reduce the pain, try using the slow breathing you learned for labor. If needed, ask your doctor or midwife about pain pills.

After birth, you'll have a lot of vaginal bleeding (called *lochia*), like a heavy period. You'll need to wear a big pad instead of a small one. You shouldn't use a tampon in the first weeks after the birth. It's normal to pass soft blood clots (like jelly), especially in the first days after the birth. Your flow is heavier and you may pass more clots in the following situations:

- when you stand up after you've been lying down
- when you have a bowel movement
- as you breastfeed

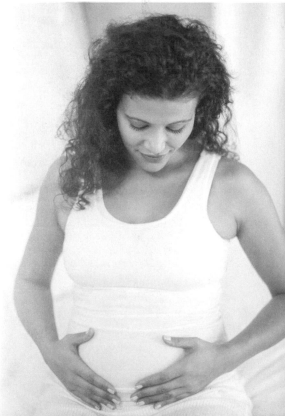

After 1 or 2 weeks, your bleeding slows down. It gradually changes from red to pink and then to tan or yellow. Your flow goes away after about 6 weeks or so. But if it increases or returns to bright red, call your caregiver.

Menstrual periods begin again about 4–8 weeks after the birth if you're not breastfeeding. If you're breastfeeding, it will take longer. Some breastfeeding mothers start their periods within a few months, though this isn't common. Some don't have a period until they start giving their baby other foods or stop breastfeeding.

You can get pregnant even if you haven't had a period yet. If you don't want to get pregnant soon, use birth control when you have sex. (See page 128 for more.)

Your Birth Canal (Vagina and Perineum)

Expect some pain if you've had stitches for a tear or episiotomy or if the vaginal area is bruised. It usually goes away in 2–6 weeks. Your stitches *dissolve* (go away) on their own in a few weeks, so they don't need to be removed.

Here are a few suggestions to help with healing and to reduce pain:

- Put an ice pack on your perineum. Put crushed ice or a frozen, wet washcloth in a ziplock bag and wrap it in paper towels. Put it inside your underwear, on top of the pad. This will hold it in place. Do this for 20 minutes, then take it off. Try to do it 2 or 3 times each day during the first few days.

- After you pee, clean yourself by pouring warm water over your perineum while you're sitting on the toilet. Or use a *peri bottle* (a squeeze bottle they give you at the hospital) to squirt the water on your bottom. Pat or gently wipe yourself dry. Wiping from front to back helps prevent infection from germs in your anus moving to your vagina.

- *Witch hazel* may provide soothing pain relief for stitches and hemorrhoids. Witch hazel pads (like Tucks) can be purchased from a drugstore. Or you can buy a bottle of witch hazel and pour some onto a few panty liners, then freeze them. Lay them on top of your larger pad each time you change it.

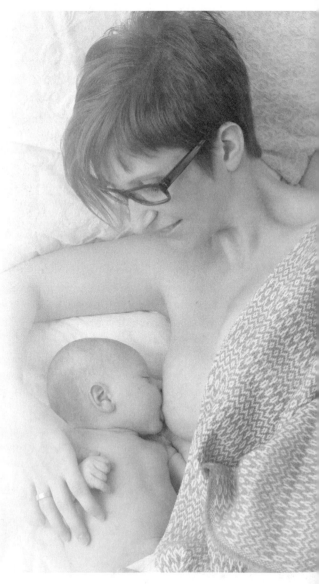

- Take a *sitz bath*. Sit in a clean tub of warm water for 10–20 minutes. You need only enough water to cover your bottom. Then get out, dry off, and lie down for 15 minutes. Lying down after your bath helps reduce the swelling in the area around your vagina. Take a sitz bath 2–4 times a day until your bottom feels better.

- Begin doing some Kegel exercises soon after the birth (see page 41). Don't be discouraged if you can't do them as well as you could before the birth. The strength of your pelvic floor muscles will improve over time.

- Lie down and rest as often as you can in the first week or two. When you sit or stand for a long time, it increases the swelling and pain around your vagina.

Maria's Story

Sitting down really hurt because I had stitches and my bottom was sore. I used witch hazel pads and ice packs. The thing that helped me most was sitting in the tub with a little warm water. I also just tried to lie down most of the time in the first few days. I spent time snuggled skin-to-skin with the baby in bed.

Your Breasts

For breastfeeding mothers: For 2 or 3 days after the birth, your breasts will produce special milk called *colostrum*. This is the only food your baby needs for the first few days. Then your milk supply will increase quickly. Most mothers say their milk "came in" when their breasts became full and hard. Let your baby nurse often or at least every 2–3 hours. This decreases the fullness and helps prevent your breasts from getting too painful (see chapter 10 for more on breastfeeding).

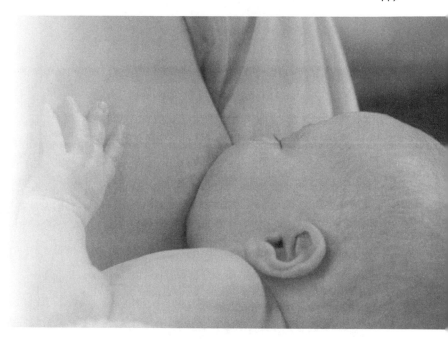

For mothers who don't breastfeed: Your breasts will probably go through the same changes as a breastfeeding mother at first. You may have a few days of heaviness and pain in your breasts. Try these methods to make you more comfortable and to stop your breasts from making milk:

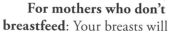

- Bind your breasts with a wide elastic bandage (like an Ace bandage), a sports bra, or a very tight bra. Wear the bandage or bra for 1–2 days starting on the second or third day after the birth. Wear it all day long, even while sleeping.
- Apply ice packs when your breasts begin to feel full and hard. Put an ice pack on top of the bandage or bra 20 minutes. Do this every 4 hours during the daytime.
- Do not breastfeed. And don't try to remove any milk from your breasts with a breast pump or by squeezing milk out with your hand. This will cause your breasts to make even more milk.
- Take ibuprofen as ordered by your doctor or midwife. This will decrease the swelling and pain.

In the past, women were given shots or pills to "dry up" their milk. These methods aren't available now because of their serious side effects. Also, they didn't work any better than the suggestions in this list.

Your Muscles and Joints

After the birth, it takes about 6 weeks for your belly muscles to regain their strength and tone. Exercise helps speed up this process (see below and page 124). If you had a cesarean birth, see page 112.

Some women feel pain in the tailbone, hips, pelvis, or lower back after the birth. Your tailbone may have been bruised when your baby came down the birth canal. If you pulled your legs very wide apart during birth, your hips may be sore for a while after the birth. Massage, baths, heating pads, and gentle exercise may help. If it's painful to walk, sit, or roll over, tell your caregiver.

Head-Lift Exercise
After pregnancy, some women notice a wide gap between their tummy muscles near their belly-button. A small gap is normal between these muscles (the *rectus* muscles). Doing this exercise helps strengthen these muscles and bring them closer together.
1.   Lie on your back with your knees bent.
2.   Cross your arms over your belly. Put your hands beside your waist.
3.   Breathe in.
4.   As you breathe out, raise your head and shoulders. At the same time, pull your hands toward your bellybutton and use your tummy muscles to pull your belly button toward your spine. 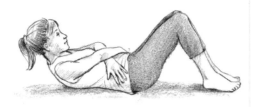
5.   Hold for a slow count of 5.
6.   Put your head down and rest for about 10 seconds.
Repeat about 20 times a day until the gap is smaller.

Your Bladder and Bowels

You may have trouble peeing because your bottom may be sore or swollen. Usually this lasts only a few days.

You may also have trouble with bowel movements after the birth. If you had an episiotomy, you may have pain from a sore bottom. Also, iron pills or pain pills can make your bowel movements harder (*constipation*). Try these suggestions to avoid constipation and help you have normal bowel movements:

- Take stool softeners. You may be given some at the hospital before you go home, or you can buy them at a drugstore. If they're ordered by your doctor or midwife, your insurance may help pay for them.
- Eat foods with fiber, such as fresh fruits, dried fruits, fresh vegetables, dark breads, cereal, beans, and lentils.
- Drink plenty of water.
- Walk and do exercises that tighten your belly muscles.
- Go to the bathroom when you feel the need to have a bowel movement. Don't wait.
- If these ideas don't help, talk to your caregiver about other medicines to relieve constipation.

Hemorrhoids (sometimes called *piles*) are painful, swollen veins in your rectum. They're common during pregnancy and more common right after birth. Hemorrhoids usually go away within a month or so after birth. Try these suggestions to decrease the pain and help hemorrhoids heal:

- avoid constipation (see page 120)
- try Kegel exercises (see page 41); these tighten the muscles in the rectum too
- try witch hazel and sitz baths (see page 118)
- if these measures don't help, talk to your doctor or midwife

Warning Signs during Postpartum
Some problems may come up after you get home. You may wonder if they're normal or serious. If you notice any of the following warning signs, call your caregiver right away:
• fever (your temperature, taken by mouth, goes up to 100.4°F or 38°C or higher)
• very heavy vaginal flow (enough to soak a big pad in an hour or less) and/or having a blood clot larger than a lemon
• stinky smell from your vagina (could smell fishy) or vaginal soreness or itching
• more pain at the site of stitches than there was the day before
• trouble peeing or pain when you pee
• sore, red, hot area on your breast, along with fever
• feeling very anxious, angry, sad, or panicky, along with trouble sleeping and eating
• sore, red, painful area on your leg (it could be a dangerous blood clot)
• pain in the bone under your pubic hair or in your lower back, along with trouble walking
• it you had a cesarean, increased pain and redness around the incision, and/or pus running out of your scar
• any new pain or sudden soreness or discomfort
• fear of abuse or violence toward you or your baby by your partner or family member

Medical Care after the Birth

You should have a checkup once or twice during the first 2 months after your baby's born. Make an appointment soon after the birth. If you wait, your doctor or midwife may be too busy to see you. Your caregiver will check your physical recovery, perineum, stitches (if necessary), and vaginal flow. If you had a cesarean birth, your scar will be checked too. Your caregiver may check your breasts and talk to you about breastfeeding. You'll also have a chance to talk about any physical or emotional problems. Talk to your caregiver about family planning. This is a good time to choose a birth control method if you haven't already (see page 128).

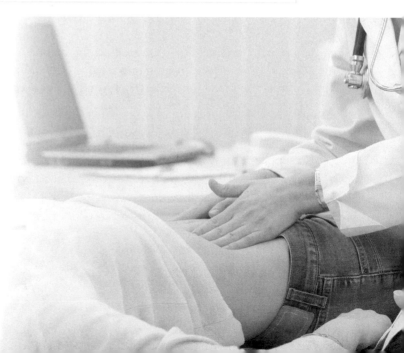

Help and Support

You may be surprised to discover how hard it is to take care of a brand-new baby, especially if it's your first one. It's a big challenge. You're recovering from pregnancy and birth, and you have to learn this new job at the same time. In addition, you aren't getting a full night's sleep or much down time because your baby needs to eat and have her diapers changed.

It's normal to need some help when you have a new baby. If you have help, you'll get used to being a parent quicker. Also, you'll have more time to sleep and rest.

Jenny's Story

Mom wanted me to stay at her place after Emily was born, so she could take care of me. I didn't want to, because I felt like I needed to be able to do everything on my own. But Kyle encouraged me to take Mom up on her offer. He had to go back to work right away, and he wanted me to have some help. I spent most of the first week lying around holding my baby. Mom treated me like a princess. It was actually pretty great, because I could focus on learning to be a parent while she took care of me. Kyle came over after work every day. He's great with Emily.

Try to say yes when people offer to help. Most people are glad when you accept their help. Some people don't offer because they don't want to get in the way. So make sure you also ask for help if you need it. Maybe your mother, aunt, or sister can stay for a while. Friends from work, church members, or neighbors may be happy to help with some things. Even an older child can help around the house. You may need help with some or all of these things:

- shopping for groceries and baby supplies
- doing laundry
- cooking
- cleaning up
- watching your baby while you nap or take a shower

Some people aren't very helpful. They make life harder for you. Sometimes they make more work for you or they upset you by not understanding what you're going through. Try to keep these people away. This is no time to entertain or get more stressed. If you don't have enough help, ask your caregivers or the hospital staff if they know of resources for help at home.

Advice to Helpers (Family and Friends)
Your support and love are important to the new mother. Here are a few helpful hints:
• A new mother needs to hear that she's doing a good job. When she does something "right," tell her.
• Offer help, especially if she can't (or won't) ask for it.
• Ask her how you can help (preparing meals, doing laundry, shopping, or cleaning).
• Don't spend all your time holding and caring for the baby, unless she can't. Take care of her so she can focus on taking care of her new baby.
• Let her take care of the baby in her own way. She may choose to do things differently than you would.
• Plan to work hard, sleep little, and leave tired! She'll appreciate all you've done.

Staying Healthy after the Birth

What can you do to feel better and recover quickly after having a baby?

Get Enough Rest and Sleep

Getting enough sleep is a big problem for new mothers and fathers. Lack of sleep slows your physical and emotional recovery. Rest can give you the energy you need to take care of yourself and your baby.

All babies need to wake up and feed at night. Some babies seem to sleep more during the day than at night. Try not to worry. Gradually your baby will need to feed less at night and will sleep longer.

Here are some helpful hints on how to get enough sleep:

- Try to sleep or rest when your baby sleeps—even during the daytime. This may seem hard if you're used to sleeping only at night.
- Think about how much sleep you usually need each day (8 hours?). That's the amount of sleep you should try to get after your baby's born. It won't be all at one time, but it can add up over the course of the night and into the day.
- Plan to stay in bed (or keep going back to bed) until you've slept enough. This means not getting up except for caring for your baby, eating meals, and making trips to the bathroom. You may have to stay in bed from 10 PM until noon the next day to get the amount of sleep you need!
- Rest or sleep before doing other things. Someone else can do the laundry and dishes. Or let these things wait until you've had a nap.
- If you're worried about not hearing your baby's cries, try keeping your baby close to you while you sleep, such as in a crib in your room. In the first weeks, babies usually sleep more when they're with their parents.
- Let others hold and care for your baby while you rest.
- If you have other children, your best chance for sleep is to have someone watch them while you nap.

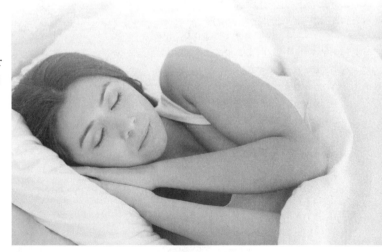

Tanya's Story

I was worried about having a 3-year-old and a new baby. It seemed that Molly needed so much from me. I didn't know how I could take care of a little baby too. Jason got only 2 weeks off from work. We were both tired and busy, but we managed. We're a pretty good team. Our friends brought us food, which was great.

Molly didn't pay much attention to the baby. Sometimes she ignored me too. I know she didn't mean it, but it hurt my feelings. She liked playing with her dad. It was tough for Molly when Jason went back to work. Even if I couldn't play as much, I could talk and listen to her while taking care of the baby. It was nice when a friend invited Molly over to her house. Molly liked playing with her kids, and I got a break.

Exercise to Help Get Back in Shape

If your labor and birth were normal, it's safe to begin doing mild exercises within a day or so. You don't have to, though. It's all right to wait. Start gradually and do what makes you feel good. Do your Kegels. Take a walk. Do some exercises that strengthen your tummy muscles.

You know you're overdoing it if the exercises make you very tired, cause pain, or increase your vaginal bleeding. If that happens, take it easy for a few days and start exercising again, but not so hard. Of course, if any of these problems remain after taking it easy, call your caregiver.

If you had a cesarean birth, your belly will be sore near the incision (the cut into your belly). You'll need to wait longer before you begin exercising. Follow your caregiver's advice about exercise and other activities such as driving, stair climbing, and lifting.

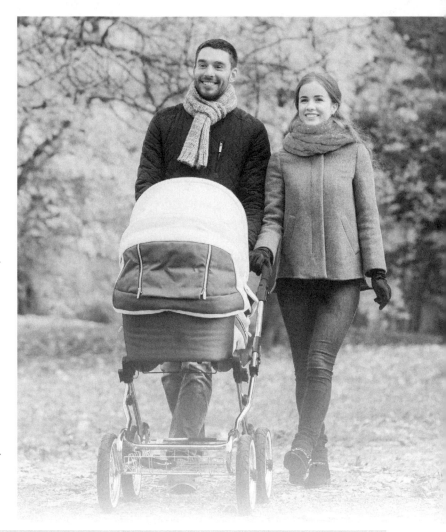

Sit-Back Exercise

A week or two after the birth, begin doing this exercise. It helps your tummy muscles get stronger.

1. Sit with your knees bent and your feet flat on the floor.

2. Hold your baby close to your chest, or rest him on your legs. (If you do this exercise without your baby, stretch your arms out in front of you.)

3. Slowly lean back about halfway to the floor. (Or stop when you begin to feel unsteady or your tummy muscles feel weak.)

4. Stay leaning back for a slow count of 5.

5. Sit back up.

As your muscles get stronger, count to 10. Then work toward doing 5 sit-backs during each exercise session.

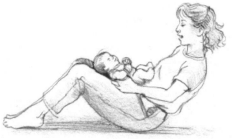

Eat Healthy Foods

Continue to eat well after your baby is born. Follow your caregiver's advice about taking prenatal vitamins and iron pills.

To lose extra pounds after the birth, you don't have to go on a strict diet. Most new mothers lose weight gradually over several months as long as they don't eat a lot more than they need. If you want to lose weight, aim to lose just 1–2 pounds per week.

If you're breastfeeding, you'll make healthy breast milk even if your diet isn't perfect. But if you eat poorly, nutrients will be taken from your body's supply to make milk. After a while, this will affect your health. So to keep feeling good when you're breastfeeding, try these suggestions:

- Eat a variety of healthy foods.
- Eat enough to maintain your weight. (You may need to eat more than you usually do.)
- Eat what tastes good.
- Drink plenty of water and other fluids. If you feel thirsty, drink something. You know you're getting enough if your pee is light yellow.

You may wonder if certain foods should be avoided. You may be told to avoid eating cabbage, broccoli, and spicy foods because they cause more gas and make your baby fussy. That's usually not true. In fact, many mothers will tell you that their babies do well when they eat what they like! Usually the foods you eat are fine for breastfeeding.

Caffeine affects sleep, but usually a small amount doesn't have much effect on a baby. If you want coffee, tea, or a cola, try drinking 1–2 cups a day and see if it makes any difference in your baby's sleep pattern or crying.

What should you *not* have when you're breastfeeding? Alcohol, the chemicals in cigarettes (such as nicotine), and other drugs, all of which go into breast milk and harm new babies. It's best to limit or avoid using them while breastfeeding. Check with your doctor, pharmacist, or breastfeeding counselor before taking any medication.

Some babies are fussy if their mothers eat very large amounts of one specific food. Try to eat normal-size servings of many different foods.

If you think a certain food is bothering your baby, stop eating it. Wait a few days and see if your baby seems better. If it doesn't make any difference, try that food again and see how your baby reacts. Also, talk to your caregiver or a breastfeeding counselor if you have questions about what to eat. If your baby develops a severe rash, diarrhea, or blood in their poop, this can be a sign of an allergy to something in your diet.

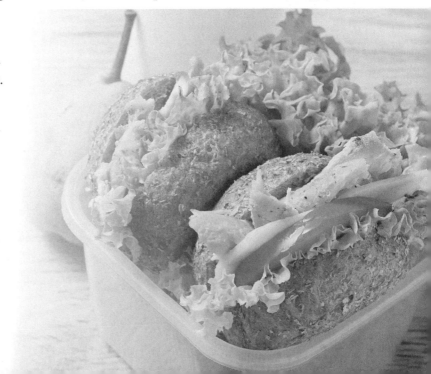

Your Feelings and Emotions

After the birth, you may be surprised at how moody you are. You may be excited, tired, and irritated—all at the same time. These ups and downs are caused by changes in your hormones—and the big life changes that come with having a baby. For most women, these feelings are mild and go away within a week or so.

Baby Blues

Baby blues are common. About 8 out of 10 new mothers have them. These are some symptoms of having the baby blues:

- You cry easily.
- You feel like you can't do everything.
- You wonder if you're a good mother.
- Sometimes you love being a parent; sometimes you hate it.

Baby blues are normal, and they're usually over within 2 weeks after birth. Here are some suggestions to help you feel better:

- Get as much sleep or rest as you can. Eat well.
- Reduce any pain that you're feeling (see pages 112 and 117–121).
- Ask family and friends to help.
- Accept that these feelings are normal and don't feel guilty for having them, or think that they make you a bad parent.
- Let yourself cry when you need to.
- Reach out to family and friends for emotional support. Don't be afraid to share your feelings.
- Get outside in natural light. Go for a walk.
- Take some time for yourself, away from chores and baby care, if you can.

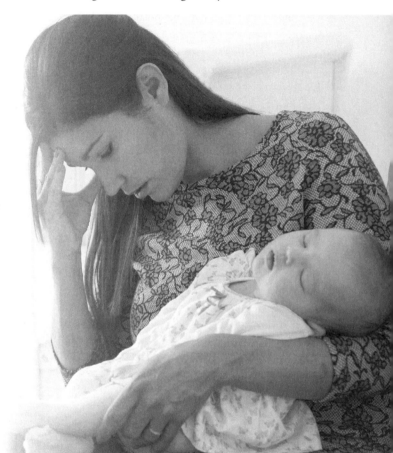

Cami's Story

The hardest thing for me was being alone all day with Tommy. Chris had to go right back to work. I got so tired. Sometimes when Tommy cried, I cried too. I loved Tommy so much. But I kind of hated being a mom. I felt like a terrible person. When I got more sleep and talked things over with my sister and Chris, I felt better. Then I wondered how I could have felt unhappy about my new life.

Postpartum Mood Disorders

Perinatal mood and anxiety disorder (PMAD) is a term used for emotional problems that occur before or after birth and are serious enough for a woman to need professional help. *Postpartum depression* is the best-known form. Some women experience prenatal depression, postpartum anxiety, and postpartum obsessive-compulsive disorder. About 2 in 10 women have a perinatal mood disorder, as do 1 in 20 new dads.

Often a PMAD begins between 6 weeks and 6 months after the birth. However, it can start anytime during pregnancy, in the first year, or when you stop breastfeeding. You may be the first one to notice the signs, or a family member might help you recognize them.

- **Signs of a mood disorder**: The symptoms are often described as "crying more than the baby cries and sleeping less than the baby sleeps." Here is a detailed list of symptoms: crying a lot more than usual
- having trouble sleeping, even when very tired, because you're worried about the baby or caught up in your feelings and thoughts
- not feeling hungry, forgetting to eat meals, or eating a lot
- not wanting to take care of yourself
- not being interested in anything, even things that would normally interest you
- sudden outbursts of being very angry and yelling at others
- having panic attacks (difficulty breathing, trouble swallowing, racing heartbeat)
- being very frightened of being left alone with the baby
- having thoughts of hurting yourself or your baby
- having flashbacks about difficult times in the past or during the birth

There are good ways to treat a PMAD, especially if you start early, including self-help, counseling, and/or medication.

What to do if you have a perinatal mood disorder:
- Realize that you're not a bad person. It's not your fault that you're having these thoughts or feelings.
- Be good to yourself by following the self-care tips we recommended for baby blues.
- Tell a trusted person how you're feeling, especially if you're worried about hurting yourself or your baby.
- Call a PMAD support hotline or attend support groups to share your feelings with others who have been through it.
- Get counseling from a therapist, ideally one who specializes in PMAD, and take medication if advised.

Finding the Support You Need

Ask your doctor, midwife, hospital, or social worker about support groups and therapists in your area. Contact Postpartum Support International via their hotline at 800-944-4773 or by visiting www.postpartum.net. They can offer support and connection to local resources.

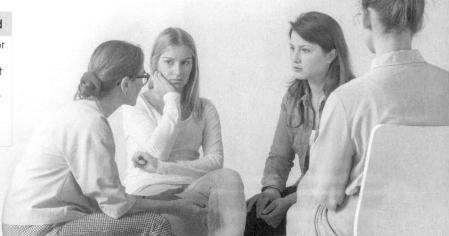

Family Planning and Sex after the Birth

Some women want to have sex soon after the birth. However, most women prefer to wait awhile. They're afraid that it'll hurt, or they're too tired. Doctors and midwives tell you to wait until your stitches are healed and your vaginal flow (lochia) is almost gone. This takes about 6 weeks. Of course, you should wait until you feel like having sex. If your partner is ready before you are, talk about it, and try to be honest and kind to each other. Don't worry that you've lost your desire for sex—it will come back.

If your vagina hurts during sex, try being on top of your partner. This puts less pressure on the back of your vagina (where stitches are done for a tear or episiotomy). Also, it's normal for your vagina to be dry after birth when you're breastfeeding. Vaginal dryness may cause pain during intercourse. You can put a water-soluble lubricant like K-Y Jelly or Astroglide into your vagina or on your partner's penis. This helps make sex more enjoyable. You can buy vaginal jelly or cream at a drugstore. But don't use ones with estrogen; they might reduce your milk supply.

If you're breastfeeding, you may leak milk when you orgasm. This is a normal effect of your hormones. Many couples take it as a positive sign that you're having a good time. But if you're uncomfortable with it, wear a bra with nursing pads during sex.

Family Planning

To give your body a chance to recover from being pregnant, try to wait at least 1 year before getting pregnant again. Remember that you can get pregnant before your menstrual periods return, because you release an egg (ovulate) two weeks *before* your first period.

Talk to your caregiver about birth control. These methods of birth control are safe to use during breastfeeding:

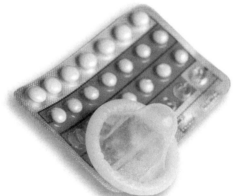

- mini-pill—a progestin-only birth control pill (pills or patches with estrogen in them affect breast milk supply)
- Depo-Provera shots
- condom along with spermicidal (sperm-killing) foam, cream, or jelly
- diaphragm or cervical cap
- IUD (a small plastic device put into your uterus during a vaginal exam)
- emergency contraception

Having a Baby Changes Your Life

Being a new parent brings a mixture of feelings—excitement, exhaustion, fear, and joy. There's nothing like it. You feel like your life has changed overnight.

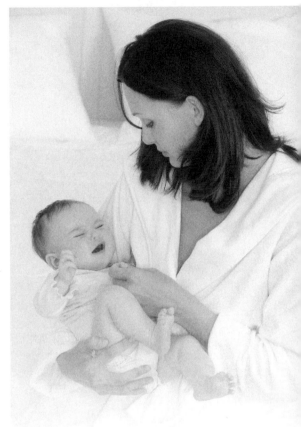

When Will I Get Back to "Normal"?

In the first few months, we expect everything to feel crazy and hard for a new family. You may find yourself desperately wishing life would get back to normal. But your life won't ever go back to your old normal. However, you *will* find a new normal: a time when you find yourself feeling as if you've always been a parent, and you can't imagine not being one. Most parents find they reach a new normal around 6 months after the birth.

It takes time to recover physically and adjust emotionally after you have a baby. The amount of time depends on some of these factors:

- your physical and mental health
- the amount of love and help you get from family and friends
- your experience and confidence with baby care
- your baby's health and personality
- your financial situation and need to return to work

If things are going well, you'll recover more quickly and adjust faster than if you're having troubles or problems.

Maria's Story

I had to take the bus when Isabel and I went to the mother-baby class. At first, I didn't want to go because it was too much trouble to get out of the house. Am I glad I went! It was so good to have other moms to talk to. It became my lifeline because my family lives so far away. All the other moms knew what I was going through. Being a new mom was tough. But when Isabel finally started smiling and cooing at me, it made up for the hard times.

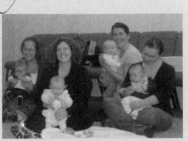

Parenting

Parenting is challenging and tiring. Yet it's one of the most important and rewarding jobs you'll ever have. The early weeks aren't easy. However, a good start helps you build a strong family.

Even if you don't know much about babies, you can learn how to be a good parent. Watch your baby. Pay attention to her behavior to find out what she wants and needs. (For more about babies, see chapter 11.)

You can also take parenting classes. Look for classes or groups for new moms or parents of young children at community colleges, hospitals, churches, or elsewhere in your community. Other parents are a great source of emotional support, parenting tips, and friendship. Contact your local health department or childbirth education agency to learn about parent support in your area.

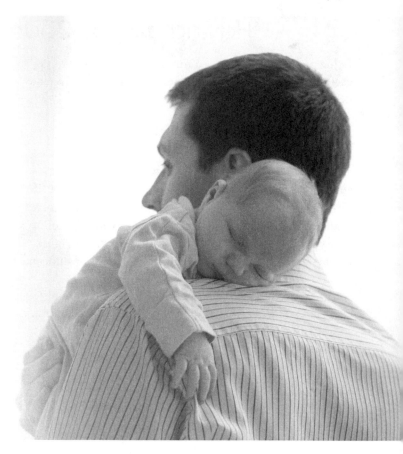

Note to Fathers and Partners

This early time with your new baby will be important for both of you. Spend some time learning about your baby and learning your own style of parenting. The baby will know your voice and will respond to you in a special way. (See page 171 for more about your role.) Caring for your new baby during these early months will give you lifelong memories. You'll be glad you shared in the work and joy of parenting.

The early months of parenting may also be hard for you, both emotionally and physically. (For new dads, 5% experience postpartum depression.) Rest when you can, eat well, and exercise to keep your energy up. Ask friends and family members to help you take care of the new mom and baby. Seek out emotional support when you need it. Talking to other new and experienced parents can be a great way to get support and practical tips.

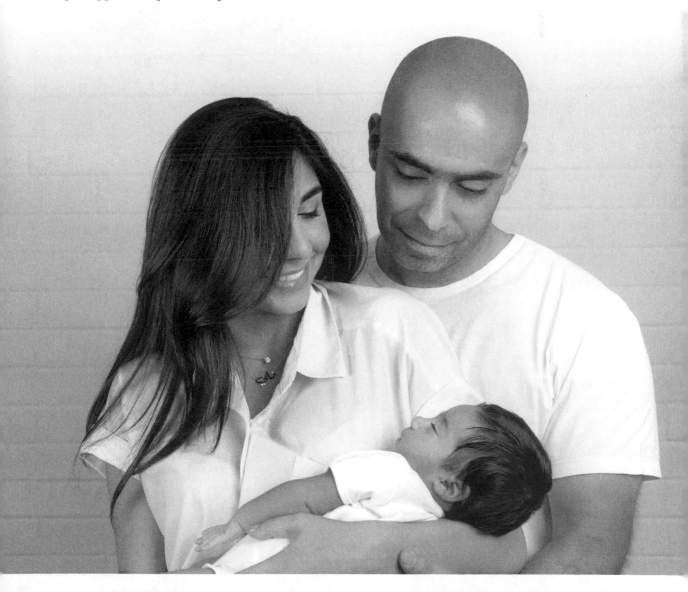

CHAPTER 10

Feeding Your Baby

During the first several months, your baby will have breast milk, formula, or both. When your baby is around 6 months old, you will start *solid foods* (baby foods) but continue with breast milk or formula till at least one year. This chapter gives you helpful hints about when and how much to feed, breastfeeding, feeding pumped breast milk, and formula feeding.

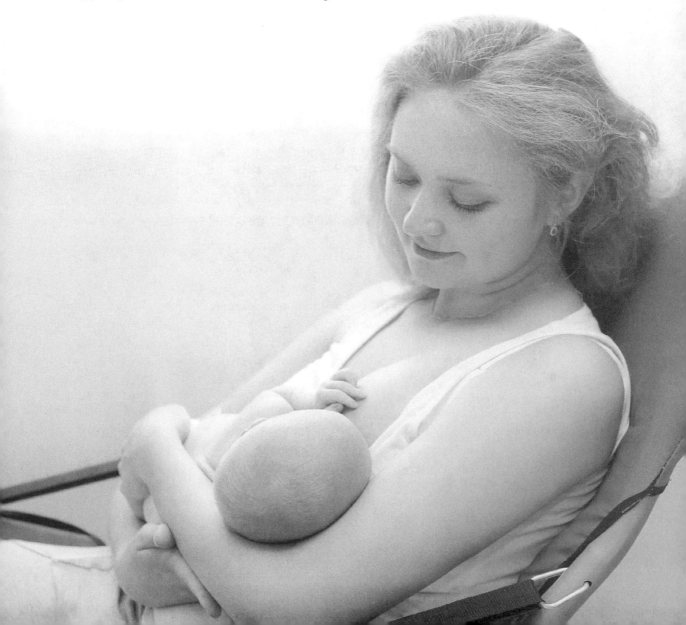

When to Feed Your Baby

Feed your baby whenever he wants to eat. He'll use hunger cues (physical signs) to tell you when he wants milk. For example, he'll suck on anything close to his mouth, like his hands, his blanket, or your arm. Or he'll make little sounds and stick his tongue out over and over, as though he's tasting the air. Or he'll turn his head side to side, looking for a nipple to latch on to. Try to feed your baby as soon as you see these cues. He shows these cues for about 10 minutes before he begins to fuss and then cry. It's harder to feed him when he's crying.

Feed your baby until he shows full cues. For example, he'll fall asleep, let go of the nipple, or slow down his sucking so he's resting much more often than sucking.

How often will your baby eat? Here are some guidelines about feeding patterns in the first 6 weeks:

- Most new babies eat every 1–3 hours. However, babies don't eat on a regular schedule. Sometimes a baby will eat every hour for several feedings and then sleep for 3–4 hours.
- Most breastfed newborns nurse between 10 and 12 times a day. Newborns who are bottle-fed may take 8 to 10 bottles a day. After several weeks, your baby will be able to take in more milk at each feeding. Then he will need to eat less often.
- Let your breastfed baby nurse at each breast for as long as he wants. Longer feedings help your baby get plenty of milk. Feedings may last 20–40 minutes or longer. If you are bottle-feeding, offer a newborn 2–3 ounces at each feeding.
- The length of a feeding often depends on your baby's age and feeding style. Some babies suck hard and fast and have shorter feedings. Others suck a little, pause, and suck again. It takes these babies a long time to get enough milk.
- In the first weeks, your baby's caregiver may recommend that you wake up your baby to feed if he sleeps more than four hours. After that, if your baby is a healthy, full-term baby, you do not need to wake him for a feeding.
- If your baby is very small, losing weight, or has jaundice, his caregiver may make different recommendations.

It's easier to feed your baby when he wants to eat rather than on a schedule. Trying to make a hungry baby wait until a certain time to eat will be upsetting for both of you. Also, it's hard to wake a baby for a feeding.

Babies have *growth spurts* at about 3 weeks, 6 weeks, 3 months, and 6 months of age. During these times, your baby is growing faster and needs to eat more often, as much as every hour or so. If you're breastfeeding, his frequent feedings tell your breasts to make more milk. When you're making enough milk, he'll go back to having fewer feedings.

These growth spurts may make you feel like you're feeding all the time. However, as your baby grows and takes more milk at each feeding, you'll begin to feel that you have more time for yourself between feedings.

Is Your Baby Getting Enough Milk?

Parents who bottle-feed their babies can easily see how much their baby is eating. (See page 147 for recommendations on how many ounces your baby should drink.)

Mothers who are breastfeeding count on certain signs to tell them that their babies are getting plenty of milk. Generally, breastfeeding mothers make plenty of milk for their babies. (If you want to increase your milk supply, see page 143.)

During the first week or so after the birth, watch for these signs that your baby is getting enough milk:

- *She actively sucks and swallows throughout the feeding.* Listen for swallowing. It sounds like an "ugh" sound.
- *She seems content after feedings.*
- *She feeds at least 8 times each day.* Most breastfed babies feed more often (10–12 times in 24 hours, for 20–40 minutes per feeding).
- In the first 5 days, *she has at least 1 wet or dirty diaper per day old.* (For example, on day 3 she should have at least 3 wet or dirty diapers, maybe more.) If she hasn't pooped in the first 24 hours of life, let her doctor know.
- After 5 days of age *she has 6–10 wet diapers each day.* If you're using disposable diapers, it's hard to tell how often your baby is peeing. If you want to be sure, you can put a small piece of paper towel in the diaper. It stays wet if your baby has peed.
- After 5 days of age, *she has at least 2–3 poopy diapers each day.* Many babies have more frequent bowel movements, often 1 after every feeding. This is fine. In the first month, it's common to see yellowish, soft poop after almost every feeding.

Your baby's weight gain tells you that she's getting enough milk. Most babies have a small weight loss right after birth. They usually are back to their birth weight by 2 weeks and double their birth weight by 4 to 6 months. Your baby's caregiver should see her in the first week or two after birth. At that visit, the doctor will weigh and measure your baby and make sure she's healthy. You may also return for a visit at the hospital or have an appointment with a public health nurse. You may want to go to your WIC clinic to check your baby's weight.

Note: Don't give your baby a bottle of water. Breast milk or properly mixed formula contains all the water your baby needs. Water can make your baby feel full so he doesn't want to nurse. This can lead to poor weight gain and jaundice.

Signs Your Baby Is Not Getting Enough Milk

Call your baby's caregiver right away if you see these signs:

- He feeds fewer than 8 times in 24 hours.
- He has dark yellow urine or he isn't peeing and pooping as much as he should be. (See above.)
- He's sleepy and not interested in feeding.
- His face, chest, and the whites of his eyes are yellowish. (Having yellow eyes is a clear sign of jaundice. Jaundice occurs when there is too much bilirubin in your baby's blood. This can happen when he doesn't get enough to eat, and he doesn't get rid of the blackish green poop that was in his bowels before he was born.)
- Anytime you're worried about your baby's feeding, contact his caregiver, a nurse, or a lactation consultant (breastfeeding expert).

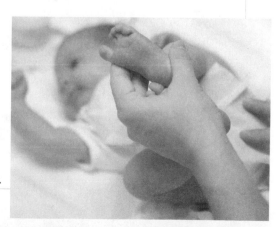

Burping and Spitting Up

If your baby is relaxed and sleepy after a feed, she may not need to burp. But, you can try just a gentle burping to be sure. If your baby is squirming, making creaking noises or seems uncomfortable during or after a feed, she probably needs to burp. Put her in a position that puts just a little pressure on her belly. Then gently pat or rub her back.

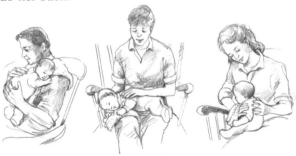

When your baby burps, she may spit up some of the milk or formula she ate. This is normal. You may be able to help her spit up less by feeding smaller amounts more often or by stopping and burping her a few times in the middle of each feeding. It also helps to hold your baby upright (sitting) after a meal, rather than laying her on her tummy or bouncing her up and down.

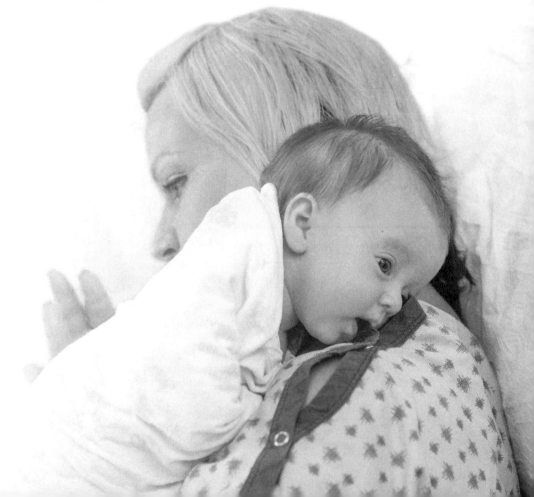

Breastfeeding

Breastfeeding is the best way to feed your baby. The more breast milk your baby eats and the more days he breastfeeds, the better, but any amount is better than none. If you're at all interested in breastfeeding, make sure you try it right after your baby is born. It's easier to start breastfeeding even if you stop a short while later than it is to never breastfeed and wish that you had.

Why is breast milk so good?

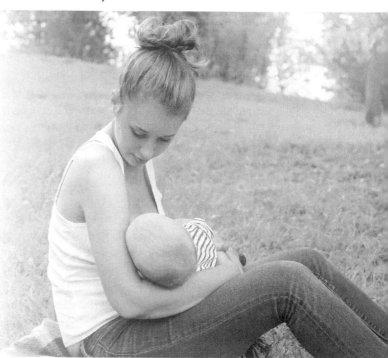

- Breast milk is the perfect food for babies. And it changes as they get older, or changes if they are sick, to give them exactly the nutrition they need.
- Breast milk is always available. And once you learn how to breastfeed, it's easier and faster than mixing formula to make a bottle.
- Breast milk is clean and safe for your baby.
- Breast milk helps your baby fight germs and sickness. Your baby will be sick less in the first year and her whole life if she is breastfed.
- Breast milk helps prevent allergies, asthma, and diabetes. Also, breastfed babies are less likely to be overweight as they get older.

Breastfeeding is also good for you. It helps reduce your risk of getting certain diseases such as breast cancer or cancer of your *ovaries*. Breastfeeding also costs less than formula. In addition, it creates a special bond between you and your baby. You'll both enjoy the closeness.

Tanya's Story

Breastfeeding was so different this time. The first time, my nipples were sore for 2 weeks and it was a real struggle, and I gave up.

This time, I wanted to breastfeed because I knew it was better for the baby, and also because my mom had breast cancer, and I wanted to do anything I could to reduce my chances of getting it.

After Michael was born, I couldn't believe how fast my milk came in. The soreness was nothing like last time. The afterpains were worse this time. Every time I fed my baby, I had bad cramps in my belly. After several days, the cramps stopped. What a relief! Then breastfeeding was easy. I'm glad I decided to do it, and I'm glad Michael will get all the benefits.

Making Breast Milk

The process of making breast milk is called *lactation*. A more common word for breastfeeding is *nursing* your baby.

Your breasts began getting ready for breastfeeding during pregnancy. By the middle of pregnancy, you began making *colostrum*. Colostrum is your baby's first milk in the days right after birth. It is thick and rich, so your baby needs only a little bit of it. Nurse frequently in your baby's first few days, because colostrum is full of nutrients, such as vitamins, protein, healthy fats, and *antibodies* (germ fighters).

After a few days, the yellowish colostrum becomes whiter, and you begin making a lot more milk. It's just the right mixture of nutrients for your growing baby. Your breasts make as much milk as your baby needs. In fact, if you have twins, you can make enough milk for 2 babies.

Although your breasts grow larger at first, they don't stay that way the entire time you're breastfeeding. They gradually get smaller when your baby starts taking other foods at around 6 months. When you stop breastfeeding, your breasts usually go back to their normal sizes.

Getting Started

The first feeding is special. It usually happens in the first hour after birth, and may be the first thing you do for your new baby. After the first couple of hours, your baby will get sleepy and won't be as interested in eating. By the second day, most babies wake up more and become eager to nurse again.

Here are some ways to make the first feedings easier:

- Hold your baby skin-to-skin for the first hour after birth. Feed your baby in that first hour when you see hunger cues.
- Have your nurse or midwife help you with the first feeding.
- Have visitors leave during the feeding if you want to be alone as you learn to breastfeed.
- Get into a comfortable position. (See page 139 for options.) Use pillows to support your arms and your baby. *Note*: you may see videos online of "the breast crawl" where the mother leans back and lays the baby on her chest and lets the baby wiggle its way up to her breast. This is a great technique for working with the baby's instincts. However, it's important that you are not lying flat on your back. That can make it difficult for the baby to breathe. Instead, sit up in a reclined (leaned back) position.

Most babies know how to nurse right from the start. Some seem sleepy or have trouble latching on to the breast. If you need help, ask your nurse or a breastfeeding specialist. With time and practice, you'll get better at it and so will your baby.

The early feedings may be different from what you expected. Your baby may only lick your breast. Or he might latch on, tug, and suck vigorously. You may be surprised at how strongly your baby suckles your nipple.

Holding Your Baby While Nursing

There are several positions you can use while breastfeeding. You may want to ask your caregiver or nurse to show you how to do them. One position may be easier in the beginning, but you'll probably use most of them at one time or another.

Before nursing, first get yourself comfortable. A nursing session may take 30 minutes, so it's important that you're somewhere that's comfortable for you. For all these positions, bring the baby up to the same height as your breast. Hold the baby close to you, so her tummy is tucked up against yours and her chin and nose are close to your nipple. Hold her so she's facing your breast, with her ears, shoulders, and hips all in a straight line, so she doesn't have to turn her head to nurse.

Cradle hold. Your baby's head rests in the crook of your arm. Your arm supports her back and your hand supports her bottom, keeping her bottom close to your belly.

Cross cradle hold. Your baby's head rests in your hand with your fingers and thumb near her neck. Your arm supports your baby's back, and your elbow keeps her bottom close to you.

Football hold. With your baby at your side, hold her head with your fingers and thumb behind her ears and your palm near her neck and shoulders. Support her back with your arm. You may place a pillow under your arm to support the baby's weight.

Lying on your side. Your baby rests on the bed next to you. Her mouth is close to your breast and her body is near your chest and belly.

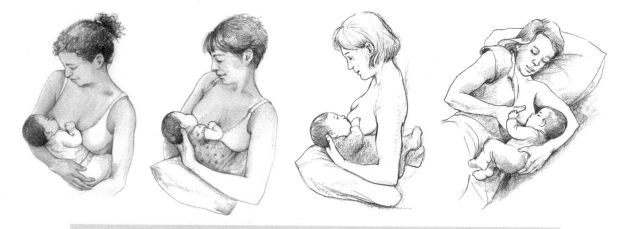

Cami's Story

I wanted to breastfeed, but I didn't think I could do it after the cesarean. I was too sore and couldn't move very well. The best thing the nurses did was to show me how to feed lying down. The nurses showed Chris how to help me. When I got home, I sat in our big easy chair and used the football hold to nurse the baby. It took about 3 weeks before breastfeeding got easier. I was proud of myself for sticking with it even though it was hard.

Helping Your Baby Get a Good Latch

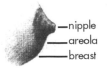

nipple
areola
breast

Latch is the way your baby's mouth holds on to your breast as he nurses. If it's a good latch, your baby gets milk, and it doesn't hurt your nipples. Some babies latch without much trouble. Others need help.

Here are some suggestions for getting a good latch. In this example, you're using the cross cradle hold:

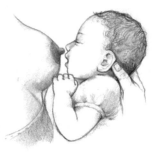

1. Bring your baby to your breast, facing your nipple, tucked close, "belly to belly."
2. Hold your baby close with your hand under his head (near his neck) and your arm against his back.
3. Some women use their other hand, support their breast. If you do this, don't lift the breast up—let it rest in its normal position. Make sure your fingers and thumb aren't in your baby's way.
4. Tilt your baby's head back just a little, place his chin on your breast, and touch his lower lip on your *areola* (the dark area around the nipple) to encourage him to open his mouth wide (like a yawn).

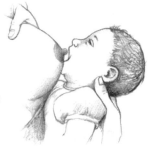

5. When his mouth is open WIDE, help him attach onto your breast. His upper lip will be over the nipple and he'll have most of your areola in his mouth near his lower jaw. This allows him to have a deep, off-center latch on the breast.
6. With a good latch, his chin presses against your breast and his nose almost touches it. (See pictures on the previous page.)
7. Let your baby suckle for as long as he likes. (Ten to twenty minutes is common.) He may come off your breast on his own. If he still wants to eat, offer your other breast.

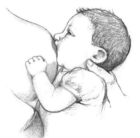

If your baby doesn't get a large part of the areola in his mouth, your nipple will probably hurt. So take him off and try again. To take your baby off your breast, slip your finger into his mouth to break the suction. Then pull him away from your breast.

Before long, you and your baby will get a good latch every time. Remember, you need to have a good latch to keep your nipples from getting sore and cracked. (See pages 143–144 for more about sore nipples.)

Maria's Story

At first, it hurt when Isabel nursed. So I asked the nurse for help. She showed me how to hold Isabel so her nose pointed at my nipple before she latched on. She said to tickle Isabel's upper lip and nose with the nipple, then wait, then tickle and wait some more until Isabel opened her mouth really wide. This helped her get more of the areola in her mouth. Not only did Isabel get more milk, the pain in my nipples went away.

Breastfeeding Basics

If you started the last feeding on your right breast, start this one on your left. By switching back and forth between breasts when you start a feeding, you make sure both breasts are making plenty of milk. (If you can't remember which side you used last time, use the breast that feels most full).

Nurse from the first breast for as long as your baby wants to suckle (usually about 10–20 minutes). When the milk flow slows down, you may notice she's swallowing less. Also, your breast feels softer when you press on it. Let your baby slide off your breast on her own.

After she stops feeding on 1 breast, burp her to help get air out of her tummy. If she fell asleep after the first breast, a diaper change may wake her for more feeding. Then offer the other breast. Let her nurse as long as she's awake and interested. If she doesn't take the second breast, don't worry.

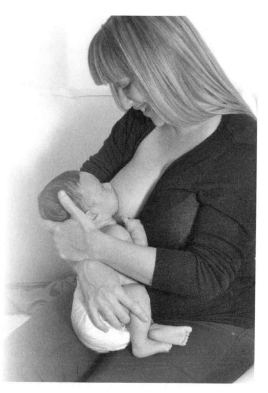

Reminder

Feed your baby anytime he shows hunger cues. For a newborn, this may be every 1 to 3 hours, or 10 to 12 times a day. The more often you nurse, the more milk you will make.

Getting Help with Breastfeeding

Most new mothers need help with breastfeeding. There are plenty of breastfeeding specialists and support groups to help you. See page 179 for contact information for the resources listed below:

- Most cities have *lactation consultants* who are trained to care for breastfeeding mothers and babies. The best lactation consultants have a certificate as an International Board Certified Lactation Consultant (IBCLC). To find an IBCLC in your area, contact the International Lactation Consultant Association (ILCA).
- Ask your childbirth educator, midwife, doctor, or nurse at the hospital. They may offer breastfeeding advice or may help you find a breastfeeding specialist.
- Contact your local WIC office or National Healthy Mothers, Healthy Babies Coalition agency.
- Call your local La Leche League (LLL) group. Going to a LLL group meeting or any group where nursing moms gather can be a great source of support and helpful tips.
- Family members and friends can also provide support and encouragement with breastfeeding.

Jenny's Story

I decided to try breastfeeding. I heard it was really good for babies. But it wasn't easy at first! I couldn't tell if I was doing it right. My mom didn't breastfeed me, so she couldn't help me much. I kept calling the clinic with questions. When Emily was about a week old, I went in and saw a lactation consultant who helps with breastfeeding. I found out I wasn't doing such a bad job after all.

Emily had lost a little weight. But the nurse said it's normal for babies to lose some weight in the first few days. She said my breasts had lots of milk, so I could stop worrying. But she also told me ways to increase my milk supply if I wanted. Mom listened to all the advice so she could help me more. After that, I took Emily in for a couple of weight checks. She kept gaining weight, and breastfeeding got easier after a couple of weeks. I'm glad I breastfed Emily. Kyle's proud of me too.

Tips for Breastfeeding Success

Almost every woman has questions about breastfeeding in the first weeks and months. The following hints may help you figure out some of your breastfeeding concerns.

Decreasing Breast Fullness/Engorgement

When your colostrum changes to milk, your breasts become heavy, full, and tender. This happens between 2 and 4 days after birth. It's normal to have some discomfort and swelling. But if your breasts become hard and painful, this isn't normal. This is called *engorgement*. When your breasts get very full, your nipples become swollen and don't stick out. This condition can make it harder for your baby to latch on.

Here's what can you do:
- To prevent engorgement, nurse often in your baby's first few days.
- To relieve breast fullness and tenderness, nurse frequently, about every 2 hours.
- To soften your nipple and areola and make it easier for your baby to latch on, try hand expressing (squeezing out) just a few drops of milk. (See page 145 for more information.) Or take a warm shower or massage your breasts with a warm washcloth to help your milk begin dripping from your breasts.
- Once your baby is nursing, use gentle pressure on your breasts to encourage milk flow. (See Encouraging Milk Flow below.)
- Let your baby nurse as long as she wants on the first breast. When she stops swallowing or falls asleep, take her off and put her on the other side. If she doesn't nurse from the other breast, hand express or use a breast pump to get some milk out of that breast.
- After nursing, apply a cool cloth or ice pack to your breasts to reduce tenderness and swelling. Some doctors and midwives suggest taking ibuprofen (a pain pill that also helps reduce the swelling).

The swollen, tender feeling usually lasts 2 days. If your baby can't nurse even after you've pumped your breasts, get help from a lactation consultant or another person who knows about breastfeeding.

Encouraging Milk Flow

Most of the time, your breasts will work just fine without extra help. But if you want to get more milk out, try putting pressure on your breast during a feeding or a pumping session to help milk flow toward your nipple.

Pressure behind the milk-producing glands (located at the outer edges of your breasts) helps with several breastfeeding problems:
- It relieves breast fullness.
- It gives your baby more milk and increases your milk supply.
- It encourages a sleepy baby to continue nursing.
- It reduces the discomfort of a plugged duct or mastitis (infected breast).

This action is sometimes called breast massage. However, don't rub in circles like you do with most massages. Instead, use one of these methods:

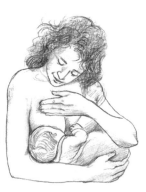

- Breast pressure: Put the palm of your hand on your ribs near the outer edge of your breast. Then slide it a little onto your breast. (Stop before you get to the areola. Pressing too close to the areola can change your baby's latch.) Press on your breast. When your baby begins to suckle less, move your hand to another part of your breast and press again. You'll notice a burst of sucking as more milk is pressed toward the nipple and into your baby's mouth.

- Breast compression: Make your hand into a C shape and cup your breast. With your palm on your ribs, put your fingers and thumb near the outer edge of your breast. Squeeze your fingers and thumb together. When your baby begins to suckle less, move your hand and compress again.

Increasing Your Milk Supply

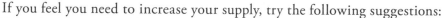

As your baby grows and gains weight, she'll need more milk. How do you increase your breast milk supply? The key is to nurse more often. You make more milk when your baby takes more milk from your breasts. This is called "supply and demand." Your milk supply naturally increases in response to your baby's demand and need for more milk.

If you feel you need to increase your supply, try the following suggestions:

- Breastfeed more often than you have been.
- Make each feeding longer. Let your baby feed for as long as she wants. If needed, switch from 1 side to the other and then back again.
- Check your baby's latch. You should be able to hear her swallowing as she feeds. If you don't hear swallowing, try again until she's latched well and you can hear her swallowing. (More swallowing means she's getting more milk.)
- Spend time snuggling in bed with your baby. This gives you time to rest and to pay close attention to her feeding cues. Have her wear only a diaper, and don't have any clothing over your breasts. Having your baby's skin touching your skin helps increase your milk supply.
- Press on your breast while feeding (as described on page 142) to increase the amount of milk your baby takes.
- Use a breast pump after feedings. Pump about 10–15 minutes per side. If your baby is unable to breastfeed, pump some breast milk and give it to her in a bottle.
- Don't give your baby formula. If she fills up on formula, it will be longer until she wants to nurse again, and she will take less milk from your breasts. This will cause your breasts to make less milk.
- Get help from a lactation consultant.

Avoiding Sore Nipples

Most new mothers have some nipple soreness during the first weeks. At the beginning of a feeding, the stretching of the nipple and areola can cause pain. It usually goes away after a minute or so when the milk begins to flow. This nipple soreness should stop after a few weeks.

Here are some ways to prevent and treat sore nipples:

- To help reduce the pain, hand express a few drops of milk to soften the areola before feeding. Try to do this before every feeding during the first week.
- Follow the suggestions on page 140 to help your baby latch on well. A poor latch is the most common cause of nipple pain. If your baby has a poor latch, correct it! The pain will go away as soon as you fix the latch.
- Feed your baby often. If you wait until your breasts are very full, it will be harder for your baby to latch on.
- Begin feeding on the less-sore side. A baby's suck is usually stronger at the beginning of each feeding.
- When taking your baby off your breast, slip your finger into his mouth to break the suction. This will help you get your nipple out of his mouth without pain.

If you have these problems, contact a lactation consultant or breastfeeding expert:
- cracked or bleeding nipples
- severe pain that continues through a whole feeding session, rather than just for the first minute or so
- pain that continues after the first month of nursing

Breastfeeding in Public

At first, you may have trouble breastfeeding without taking off your shirt and bra. After a few weeks, breastfeeding will be easier, and you'll be able to keep your clothes on. Then you'll be able to breastfeed your baby when you go out. If you're concerned about breastfeeding in front of others, here are some ways to feel more comfortable:

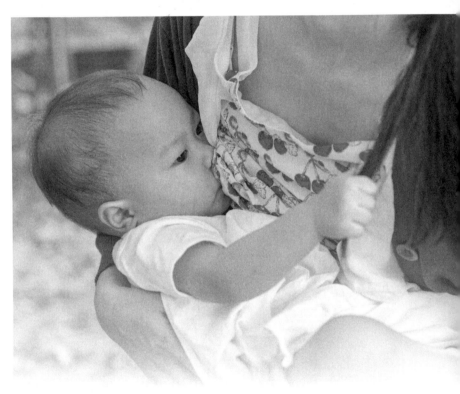

- Wear a nursing bra that unhooks above the breast. This will allow you to lower the flap without taking off your bra.
- Wear a loose-fitting shirt. Instead of undoing buttons at the top of your shirt to expose your breast, you may find it easier to lift your shirt up from the waist. When you hold your baby, she covers the bared belly.
- Take along a small blanket or shawl to put over your shoulder and cover your baby and breast.
- Practice feeding in front of a mirror. You'll see what others see when you breastfeed. When you're sure your breast is covered, you'll be more comfortable feeding in front of others.
- Try feeding in front of a friend, another breastfeeding mom, or a family member at first. When that feels comfortable, you'll be ready to feed in public situations.

Having Support for Breastfeeding

It's very important to have the support of your partner or a family member. You're more likely to succeed at breastfeeding if the person living with you encourages your efforts. To increase your chances of breastfeeding for as long as you want to, find people who are enthusiastic about breastfeeding. Talk with them as much as possible in the first weeks after the birth. With help and support, learning to breastfeed is easier. And the challenges don't seem so hard to handle.

Note to Fathers and Partners

Having a partner's support helps a mother achieve her goals for nursing the baby. Here are some things you can do: Attend a breastfeeding class with the mom during pregnancy and read this chapter so that you know more about breastfeeding and how to help her succeed. When she's worried or discouraged, you'll have great tips to offer her. When she's nursing, help her by bringing pillows, a glass of water, snacks, or something to entertain her. (Or even better, hang out together and keep her and your baby company!) Also, take on more than your share of all the other baby care jobs, such as diapering, bathing, laundry, and more.

Pumping and Storing Breast Milk

Breastfeeding milk from the breast is best for your baby and easiest for you (once you get the hang of it). But you may want or need to give your baby pumped milk from a bottle; for example, if you have a preterm baby who can't nurse from the breast, if you're returning to work or school, or if you just need a break from breastfeeding.

If you only occasionally need to collect milk, you may use hand expression. Most mothers use a breast pump. Pumping or hand expressing becomes easier with practice. It may take a while to learn how to do it effectively.

It's usually best to wait to start pumping, and wait to introduce a bottle, until your baby is breast-feeding well, which is usually about 3–4 weeks after the birth.

Hand Expression

Here's how to hand express your breast milk:

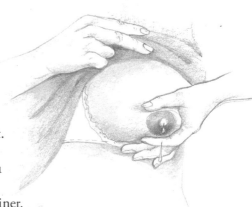

- Place your thumb on the top edge of your areola, and your fingers on the bottom edge.
- Lift your breast with your fingers.
- Gently press your breast toward your chest. Squeeze your breast between the pads of your thumb and fingers. Squeeze for 5–10 seconds until the milk stops dripping or squirting out.
- Move your fingers and thumbs to a new position, press your breast against your body, and squeeze again. Repeat until you have the milk you need.
- Collect your milk in a measuring cup or another clean container.
- At first, you may get only a few drops. With practice, you'll get a steady spray.

Pumping

If you want to buy a breast pump, check with your insurance to see what is covered. Learn more about how to choose a breast pump at http://www.kellymom. com. To learn how to use it, follow the instructions in the manual, look at the manufacturer's website, or ask someone who knows about breastfeeding.

Try pumping after a feeding. Choose a feeding when you have the most milk. Pump for 10–15 minutes per side. At first, you won't get much milk. However, after a few days of pumping at that same time, you'll get more. You will be able to pump more milk if you are calm, relaxed, in a private place, and thinking about your baby while you pump.

You'll notice that the milk changes as you go through a feeding. Sometimes it looks like nonfat milk—thin and a little bit blue. Sometimes it looks like cream—thick and yellow, with lots of fat. This is normal.

Storing Breast Milk

When you express milk, be sure your hands, pump, and storage containers are all clean. Breast milk can be stored in clean glass or plastic bottles or feeding bags that are made to store breast milk. How long can you keep your expressed breast milk?

Guidelines for storing fresh milk:
- a maximum of 8 hours at room temperature (60–85°F) OR
- 8 days in the refrigerator OR
- 6–12 months in a freezer that keeps ice cream hard

This is total storage time. If the milk was at room temperature for 4 hours, you can't then put it in the refrigerator for 8 days. You used up half its "lifespan" at room temperature for 4 hours, so only keep it in the refrigerator for half the time—up to four days.

Label the bottle or container with the date you expressed the milk. Use fresh milk first, then the oldest frozen milk next. If frozen for over 3 months, breast milk loses some nutrients and antibodies to fight infection. Still, it's far more nutritious than formula.

For directions on warming a bottle, and thawing frozen breast milk, see page 147. After thawing milk, use it right away. Or keep it for only 24 hours in the refrigerator. Don't refreeze it.

Using a Bottle

You may want to use a bottle to feed your baby pumped breast milk or formula. There are several different brands of bottles, liners, and nipples on the market. Buy 1 each of 2 or 3 different kinds and see which work best for you and your baby.

Always use clean bottles and nipples. If your water is safe to drink, you don't need to sterilize the bottles. (*Sterilizing* means boiling the bottles to get rid of germs.) Bottles may be washed by hand or in the dishwasher. Clean the nipples by hand with hot soapy water. Rinse with hot water and let them air-dry.

When preparing to feed, fill the bottle with as much breast milk or formula as you think your baby will eat at that feeding. Ask your baby's doctor for recommendations on how much to feed. A general rule of thumb is that in a 24-hour day, a baby needs to drink 2 to 2½ ounces for every pound he weighs. So if your baby is 10 pounds, he would need 20 to 25 ounces total in a day. If your baby only eats from bottles, and you gave a bottle 10 times a day, you would want about 2½ ounces at each feeding. If you breastfeed most of the time and just give 1 bottle, try giving that same 2½ ounces. If your baby still seems hungry after taking that bottle, you can offer a little more.

Babies prefer milk that is body temperature, and they get more nutrients from warm milk than from cold. To warm a bottle, put it in a bowl of water. The water should be hot but not boiling. As the water cools, add more warm water. (*Note*: if you're thawing frozen breast milk, you'll use this same method, but you'll need to keep adding in warm water till the milk is thawed, then warm.) Never warm breast milk or formula in the microwave or in a pan on the stove. Overheating may burn your baby's mouth. Also, overheating your breast milk takes away some of its special qualities.

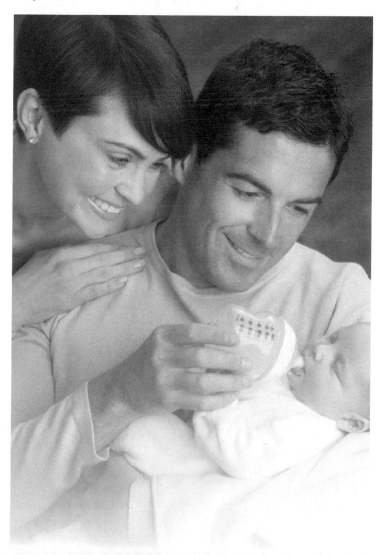

When you think the milk is warm, check the temperature by dripping a little milk onto your wrist. It should feel warm, not hot. As your baby grows older, he may like his milk a little cooler. (At any age, if you're out and about, you can feed your baby room temperature breast milk.)

If you're feeding breast milk, you may notice that the fat has floated to the top of the bottle. Gently swirl it to mix the fat in.

Tips for Bottle-Feeding

Bottle-feeding can be enjoyable for you, your baby, and your partner. Try these simple suggestions:

- Hold your baby with her head resting in the crook of your arm (just like breastfeeding). This closeness during feedings helps you and your baby develop a special bond of love.
- Never prop a bottle and leave your baby alone for feedings. She could choke if she's left alone with a bottle.
- Hold your baby sometimes in your right arm and sometimes in your left. Your baby will look at you when she feeds. Changing sides helps her eyes and neck muscles develop normally.
- Burp your baby about halfway through the feeding. As your baby grows older, she'll be able to burp on her own.
- In the first few days, feed about every 2–3 hours (or 8–12 times per day). As your baby grows older, she'll take more at each feeding and eat less often.
- Trust your baby to "tell" you how much she needs to eat. She'll probably drink more at some feedings and less at others. When she seems full, stop feeding. Don't try to get her to empty every bottle. If she quickly takes all the milk at each feeding, add another ounce of breast milk or formula to her bottle.

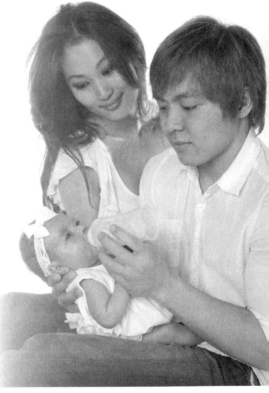

- If your baby doesn't empty the bottle, throw out any unused breast milk or formula. Also, use a clean bottle for each feeding. Germs can grow in the breast milk or formula and make your baby sick.
- Don't add cereal to her bottle—even if you heard it will get her to sleep longer. It won't. Babies shouldn't eat cereal until they're at least 4–6 months old. And when a baby starts eating cereal, it's time to learn the new skill of taking food from a spoon.
- Don't give your baby extra water. Babies don't need extra water until they begin eating solid foods. Also, don't put juice or sugary drinks into a bottle. Your baby needs breast milk or formula to grow and be healthy.

Tanya's Story

I wanted to breastfeed with Molly, but it was hard at first. And Molly cried all the time. Jason told me I should just give her a bottle. I didn't have anyone to help me. So I just quit breastfeeding and started using formula. I wish I'd called the clinic for help. The nurse said that if I'd called earlier, she would have helped me get a breast pump. Then Jason could have given her a bottle of breast milk while we worked on breastfeeding.

Figuring out how to bottle-feed took a while. I always wanted Molly to finish the whole bottle. I didn't want to waste it. But at the clinic they told me that when she stops, she's done. They were right. After that, I relaxed and then bottle-feeding was easier.

Formula Feeding

For the first 6 months of life, your baby should only drink breast milk or iron-fortified infant formula. Around 6 months, you will start adding solid foods, but breast milk or formula is still important for the first year. Other milk, such as whole milk, 2% milk, goat milk, or mixtures you make from evaporated milk or other ingredients, are not good for babies. They don't have the right mixture of vitamins, minerals, and nutrients.

Most infant formulas are made from cow milk or soybeans. If your baby is healthy and not allergic to cow milk, the best choice is an iron-fortified cow milk formula. If you want your baby on a vegetarian diet with no animal protein, you might choose a soy formula with iron. Soy formulas are also good if a baby can't digest milk sugar. This very rare condition is called *galactosemia*, and it's detected by a blood test.

If your baby has a milk allergy, his doctor may suggest a *hypoallergenic* formula (one that doesn't cause an allergic reaction). This type of formula costs more than other formulas. Examples of these formulas are Nutramigen and Alimentum.

Some parents think that an iron-fortified formula causes constipation and gas, but it doesn't. Also, babies who are fed a low-iron formula are at risk for *anemia* (not enough iron in their blood). Anemia can cause problems with your baby's brain and body development. Make sure the formula you choose has iron in it. It might not be listed on the front label, but should be included in the ingredient list.

Preparing Formula

Formula comes in various forms that are equally nutritious:
- *Ready-to-feed*. This costs the most, but it's the easiest. It's useful for trips or when you're very tired.
- *Liquid concentrate*. This requires careful mixing and takes more time.
- *Powdered formula*. This costs the least and weighs much less, which helps if you have to carry your groceries home from the store. However, it requires careful measuring and mixing. It's useful for trips if clean, warm water is handy.

When preparing formula, carefully follow the directions on the can or package. Always use the correct amount of water when mixing formula. Using too little or too much water could make your baby sick. If your water is safe for drinking, use tap water to mix the formula. If not, boil the water first. You could also use bottled water, although there's no need to, but don't use distilled water. It doesn't have the good minerals found in water. Once you have opened the container of ready-to-feed formula or have mixed up concentrated or powdered formula, you need to store it properly. If it's kept at room temperature, you should feed it to your baby within 2 hours. If you refrigerate it, you should use it within 48 hours.

Conclusion

Feeding your baby is more than just giving food. It's a wonderful time to watch and learn about your baby. When you respond to his need for milk, he learns that he can trust you. Feeding time also offers him a chance to be close to you and show his love. Enjoy this time with your baby. It'll be over before you know it.

CHAPTER 11
Caring for Your Baby

Taking care of a newborn baby may seem hard at first. It's true that babies are quite helpless. They can't use words to tell you what they need, and they can't do very much for themselves. But if you think about what few simple things your baby really needs, it's easier to figure out. Your baby needs to be fed, kept warm and clean, and cuddled and soothed when she cries.

As much as you can, try to relax and enjoy your new baby. Over time and with experience, you'll learn the best ways of caring for your baby.

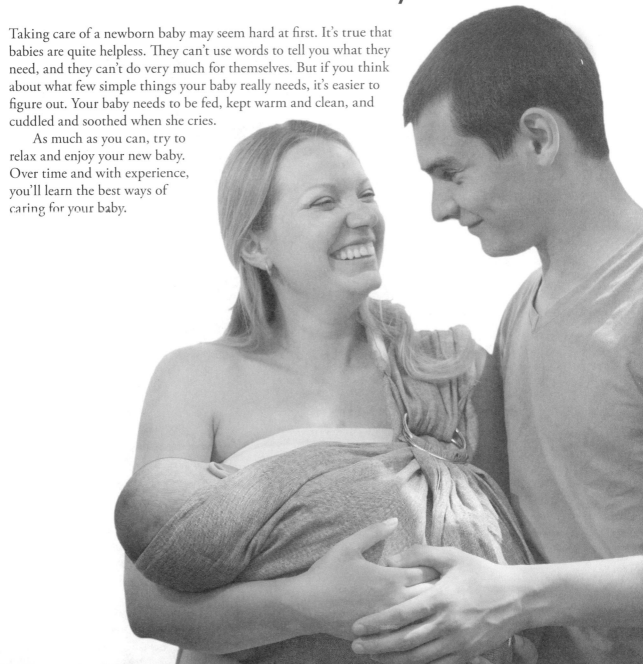

Learning about Your Baby

Until you have a baby, you might think all babies are alike. But, in fact, each baby is one of a kind. Your baby looks different and responds differently than other babies. Soon you'll learn how to respond to your individual child.

How Will Your Baby Look?

At first, your newborn baby's body will seem small, and his head will seem large. Some babies have a "cone head" because their heads changed shape to fit through the birth canal. It will return to a normal shape within a few days.

Most babies have a white, creamy substance called *vernix* on their skin right after birth. The nurse wipes most of this off, but some may remain in the folds of the skin, which is good for your baby. Your baby may have milia (small white dots) on his face, or a pimple-like rash, or "stork bites" (red marks). If your family is of Native American, Asian, or African descent, your baby might have Mongolian spots (black and blue areas on the lower back or buttocks.) These will all fade in time.

Your baby's breasts and genitals may be swollen right after birth due to your pregnancy hormones.

You may notice that your baby breathes much faster than you. He may breathe in an irregular rhythm—faster, then slower. In his sleep, he may grunt, pant, or sigh.

Most new parents have moments where they notice something about their baby, and they wonder if it's normal. In those first few days after the birth, keep a list of all those questions. Whenever your nurse, doctor, or midwife checks on you and the baby, you can ask about these things. Usually you'll learn that it's all normal for a newborn.

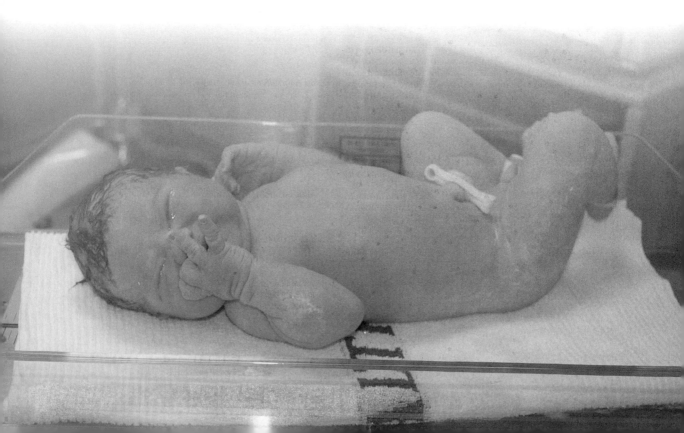

Your Baby's Abilities

For years, we thought babies couldn't do much. We believed they weren't able to tell us anything. We were wrong. Newborn babies are amazing.

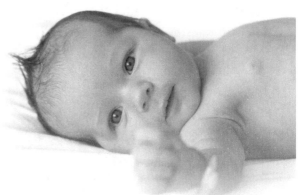

Here's what your new baby wants you to know about her:

- *She can see you clearly if you're close to her.* She loves to look at your face. Babies are sensitive to bright lights. They usually open their eyes better when lights are turned down.

- *She can hear and respond to sounds.* She may know your voice and your partner's voice. And she'll pay more attention to high-pitched voices. She may calm down when she hears sounds that remind her of being inside the womb (like the sounds of a dishwasher, vacuum cleaner, when you make a loud "shhhh" noise, or the familiar sound of a heartbeat).

- *She has a very good sense of smell and taste.* She knows your smell. The smell of your milk makes her want to suckle. Babies like the slightly sweet taste of breast milk. When you eat certain foods (such as garlic), it changes the flavor of your milk and helps to introduce your baby to flavors that you like to eat.

- *She loves to be touched.* She enjoys being held, stroked, and cuddled. She likes to be warm, but not too hot. Most new babies like to be wrapped tightly in a blanket. This is called *swaddling*.

- *She likes movement.* It reminds her of being inside you. She enjoys being rocked, swayed, or gently bounced.

Jenny's Story

Right after she was born, Emily would stare at us with big, wide open eyes. If Kyle talked to her, she'd turn and look at him. It was like she knew his voice. If he made faces at her, like sticking out his tongue or looking really surprised, she'd make the same faces. She seemed to really like it when we talked to her. So I started talking to her about everything, like how cute she was or what I was doing. I took her to the store and talked to her about what we saw there and showed her fruits and vegetables. I can tell she's done playing when she yawns or turns away or pushes my hands away.

Your baby has several normal *reflexes*. She'll cough, sneeze, yawn, and hiccup. Many reflexes are reactions to something that happens to her. She grabs your finger when you place it in her hand. She jumps at a loud noise or quick movement. You'll notice that when she's on her back, she startles easily, throwing her arms out as if she's trying to catch herself from falling. This often happens when you are calming her or when you try to lay her down to sleep, and the startle wakes her back up. It can help to swaddle her (see page 159) or hold her on her side or stomach instead of her back. When you lay her down in her crib, lower her down on her side first, then gently roll her onto her back to sleep.

Cues: How Your Baby Tells You What He Needs

At birth, your baby can let you know what he wants, likes, and doesn't like. He does this by showing you *infant cues*. As you get to know your baby better, it'll be easier to understand his cues.

Crying may mean almost anything. It may be his way of saying he's hungry, tired, lonely, uncomfortable, or overstimulated. Luckily, your baby usually gives you several gentle hints before he starts crying. Crying is a late cue, which means he uses it only when the gentle hints didn't work. Try to notice other ways he tells you what he needs.

- Hunger cues: Turning toward your breast (called *rooting*), sticking out his tongue, sucking motions, or sucking his hand tells you he's ready to eat. He may also make "enh" or "neh" sounds.
- Tired cues: Drooping eyelids, glazed eyes, yawning, and rubbing his eyes tell you he's tired and may need to sleep.
- Poop cues: Grunting, clenching his fists, pursed lips, or a serious expression as though he's thinking hard may all show he's getting ready for a bowel movement. Holding him in a sitting position may help him to get the poop out.
- Temperature cues: If he's too hot, he may be sweaty, flushed, or breathing faster than usual. If he's too cold, his skin might look mottled (pale or bluish splotches on his skin).
- Playtime cues: When he is relaxed and opens his eyes wide and stares at you, he wants you to look at him. If you talk or sing to him, or smile at him, you'll see his face light up. When he's about 6 weeks old, he'll begin smiling at you. When your baby makes sounds or coos, he's trying to talk to you. He loves it when you make the same sounds back. Babies have an amazing ability to help their parents fall in love with them.
- Break-time cues: If he stiffens, pushes his hands toward you as if trying to push you away, turns away, or stops looking at you, even when you're trying to get his attention, he may need a break. Babies get tired quickly, even when they're having a good time. If he gets fussy when you're playing, slow down a bit. Just relax and hold him quietly without looking at him. After a break, he'll show playtime cues when he's ready for more fun.
- Overstimulated cues: A grunting, grinding cry that turns into high-pitched screams tell you that you did too much, and he is overstimulated. If this happens, try one of the soothing techniques on page 161. An example would be swaddling your baby and gently rocking him while you hum. Whatever method you choose to try, try it for at least five minutes before switching to a new one. Changing from one activity to another will just stress your overstimulated baby more.

Tanya's Story

I didn't know about baby cues when I had Molly. It seemed to me that she was perfectly happy, then suddenly screaming. But now when I look back at videos of her, I can see she was trying her best to tell me what she needed.

But with Michael, most of the time, I could tell what he wanted. He really let me know when he was ready to eat. He started sucking on anything in sight, like his hand or my cheek. Once he even started sucking on his dad's nose! When Michael finished nursing, he would look milk drunk. Then he would get this really funny expression on his face. He'd raise up his eyebrows until his forehead wrinkled, make his mouth into a little O shape, and then grunt. Then you'd hear this big pooping sound!

Your Baby's Personality

Your baby's size and abilities will change quickly. However, her basic nature won't change very much as she grows older. Each baby has her own personality, also called *temperament*. Some babies are very active; others are mellow. Some babies are very regular—they sleep, eat, and poop at the same time every day. Some do not. Some startle very easily; others stay calm in all situations. When you watch other children, you'll notice these differences.

Other parents may offer you lots of advice for how to care for your baby. You can try the suggestions that sound good to you. But if it doesn't work for you, that doesn't mean you're doing something wrong. What works for other babies may not work for your baby. Your child will be like a puzzle. It will take time to figure her out. But eventually, if you tune into your unique baby and her needs, you will know your child better than anyone else does.

Some babies are more challenging than others. These babies are very active, have intense reactions, and irregular eating and sleeping patterns. With this type of baby, it may take more time and special soothing methods to make her comfortable or help her go to sleep. Also, you may need help from family and friends with this *high-needs* baby. Staying calm, having familiar routines, and always responding to her in the same way will help her settle down.

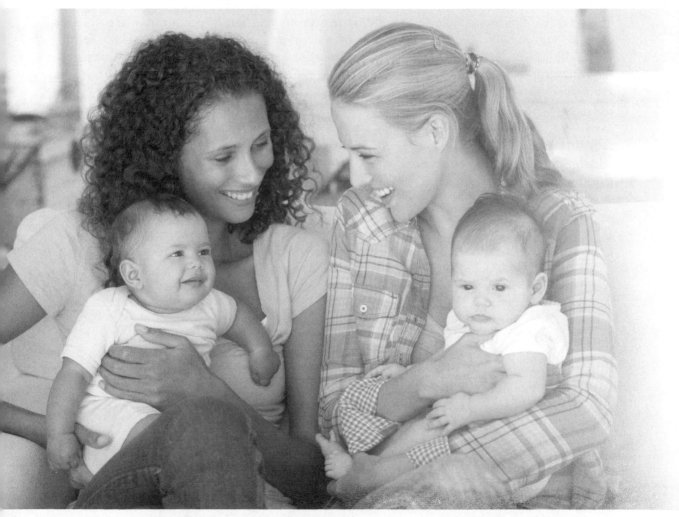

Your Baby's Daily Care

You may be surprised at how busy you are taking care of your new baby. You may get frustrated when you think about how little time you have to do anything else. It helps to remember that most new mothers feel this way. This section describes the many things you and your baby will be doing each day.

Diapering Your Baby

Babies pee and poop often. A baby's bowel movements (BMs) are different from an adult's. During the first day or so, your baby's poop (called *meconium*) will be blackish green and sticky. By the third or fourth day, your baby's poop will be runnier and yellowish. Doctors and nurses often use the term *stools* when talking about your baby's BMs or poop.

The number and type of poopy diapers depend on the type of milk your baby gets. Breastfed newborns usually have runny yellow stools after most feedings (as many as 8–12 each day). Formula-fed newborns usually have pasty, light yellowish brown stools several times a day. As your baby gets older, he'll poop less. Your baby will pee (urinate) often.

You need to change your baby's diaper every time he poops. You can use cloth or disposable diapers.

- Cloth diapers can be washed at home, or you can use a diaper service. (If you want to wash your own, search online for great suggestions from parents who have figured out how to make this as easy as possible.) You cover the cloth diaper with waterproof pants or diaper wraps to keep your baby's clothes dry. Diaper wraps use Velcro to hold the diaper in place. With waterproof pants that have an elastic waistband, you'll need diaper pins, clips, or fitted diapers that snap shut.
- Disposable diapers come in a variety of sizes and styles. They have Velcro-like tabs to hold the diaper in place. Disposable diapers are easy to use, but they cost more than washing your own diapers.

Here's how to keep your baby's bottom clean and avoid *diaper rash*:

- Change your baby's diapers whenever he poops or has peed a lot. This is usually every 2 or 3 hours.
- Clean your baby's diaper area well at each diaper change. Use a diaper wipe or a washcloth with mild soap and water.
- When it's easy to do so, let your baby's bottom air-dry a little before putting a new diaper back on.
- If your baby develops diaper rash, try these tips:
  - If you wash your own diapers, use a detergent with no perfumes and dyes, and rinse them twice.
  - If you use disposables, switch to a different brand to see if it's less irritating.
  - Put a soothing cream or ointment on your baby's bottom when it's clean and dry. Avoid ones with zinc oxide. Zinc oxide is very hard to clean off and is bad for your local water supply. Ask other parents for recommendations. Some ointments work great; others do not.
- Baby powder isn't recommended because the powder goes into the air and may hurt your baby's lungs.

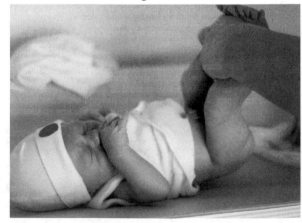

To learn how to change a diaper, ask any experienced parent to show you. In newborn care classes, there is often a chance to practice diapering a doll.

Bathing Your Baby

Newborn babies need to be kept clean, but they don't need a bath every day. Anytime you want to (or your baby needs it), you can give her a sponge bath. This just means taking a warm, wet washcloth and wiping your baby's skin clean. You can do her whole body or only the parts that need it. You can also give a tub bath, either by putting her in a special baby-size bathtub or in the sink, or by taking her into the big bathtub with you. (Get your partner to help with this. When you're done with the bath, it's much safer for you to hand the baby to another adult to dry off than it is for you to try to climb out of the wet, slippery tub with that wet, slippery baby.)

When giving your baby a bath, check the temperature of the water first by testing it with your elbow or the inside of your wrist, which may be more sensitive to temperature than your hand is. It should be comfortably warm, but not too hot. If you use soap, choose a mild one without a lot of

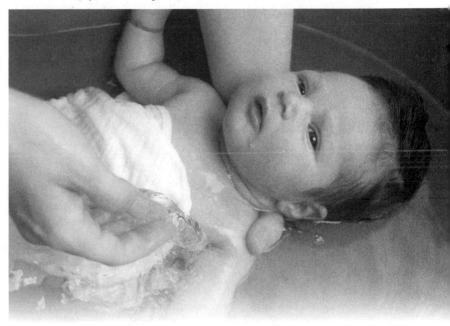

perfumes. Your baby will enjoy bath time more if you make sure the room is warm and not drafty, and wrap your baby up in a warm towel after the bath.

For lots of tips on how to bathe a baby, search on You-Tube or elsewhere online. Try to choose websites that are written by trained experts who have worked with many families, not people who have only parented one or two. You will likely find lots of good advice on the Internet, but you may also find some bad advice. If you're not sure about something you find, ask an experienced parent or your baby's caregiver.

Jenny's Story

I never thought baby care would be a problem. I used to babysit, so I thought I had it figured out. But those babies were a lot bigger than a newborn! Emily was tiny. The nurse in the hospital showed us how to hold Emily and how to swaddle and diaper her. At home, Mom showed us how to give a bath. We cleaned the kitchen sink and filled it several inches deep with warm water.

We put a folded towel in the bottom of the sink to keep Emily from sliding around. I kept my arm under her head and held her arm the whole time. Mom showed us how to lay a washcloth on her chest to keep her warm while she was kicking in the water. When we took her out, we learned to quickly wrap her in a baby towel to keep her warm. Emily really likes bath time. We only do it when she's rested, fed, and calm. If we tried when she was tired or hungry, I think she'd melt down.

Cord Care

Shortly after the birth, a plastic clamp is put on the umbilical cord, and the cord is cut, leaving about 1–2 inches of cord. The clamp probably will be taken off before you leave the hospital. If not, you can go back to the hospital or to your doctor's clinic and have it taken off. As the cord dries, it gets harder and shorter and turns black. It usually falls off between 1 and 2 weeks after birth. Cord care is done to keep the area clean and dry, and to prevent infection.

- Clean the cord daily or whenever it gets dirty from bowel movements. Use a cotton swab and warm water to clean around the base of the cord.
- Allow the cord to air-dry. Or dry it well using a cotton swab.
- To keep the cord clean and dry, fasten the diaper below the belly button area until the cord falls off.
- Call the doctor if the cord smells bad, if the skin near the cord is red, or if you see pus or bright red blood. (It's normal to see a little dark red blood or clear yellow fluid as the cord falls off.)

Your family might recommend drying agents (like rubbing alcohol) or home remedies for cord care. Most are not needed, and some may be dangerous.

Dressing Your Baby

Babies are messy. Some days your baby can make it through the day in 1 outfit; some days you might need to change his clothes 5 or 6 times. Your baby will probably spit up a little milk after he feeds. Also, pee and poop may leak out of his diaper. Try to have enough clothes so you have to wash his clothes only every few days. (*Tip*: Try shopping for baby clothes at thrift stores and consignment shops or look on Facebook for local groups like "Buy Nothing," where people give away used items. You'll find great deals, and usually the baby clothes are still in good shape.)

When dressing your baby, a good rule of thumb is to dress him in slightly warmer clothing than you are wearing. So if you're wearing a short-sleeve shirt, he would wear a long-sleeve shirt. If you're wearing a sweater, you might put him in a warm sleeper and add a hat to keep his head warm. Keep the temperature in your home set to a temperature you find comfortable. Don't overheat the baby by turning the heat up high.

Never leave your baby alone when changing his clothes or diaper. He may fall off the changing table, counter, or bed. Before you start to dress him, have all his clothes nearby so you won't need to reach and risk taking your hand off him. Some changing tables have straps to hold the baby, but you can't rely on them to prevent a fall.

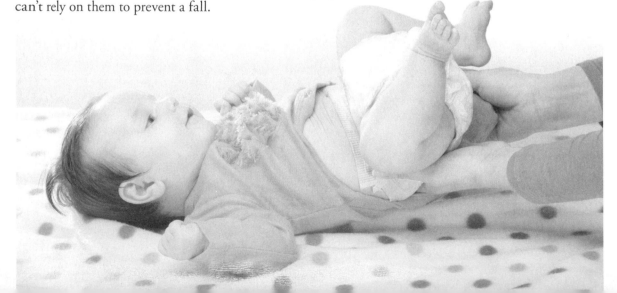

Swaddling

When you're getting ready to soothe a tired baby to sleep or when you want to calm a crying baby, a great first step is to swaddle her. To swaddle a baby, wrap her up tight in a lightweight blanket. Your nurse or midwife can show you how to do this, or you can search on YouTube for videos of swaddling. (For older babies who can escape a regular swaddle, search for videos on how to double swaddle.)

Swaddling calms many babies immediately, but it can seem to upset other babies. (Partially because you have to lay a baby on her back to swaddle her, and some babies cry more when they're on their backs than when you hold them on their sides or stomachs.) Even if your baby doesn't calm down right away when you swaddle her, it's still a helpful first step. Once you do soothe your swaddled baby, the swaddling will help her stay calm by preventing her from startling.

Swaddling also helps a baby sleep for longer stretches than she would if not swaddled. However, it's important to remember that a swaddled baby should be put down only on her back, never laid down on her tummy to sleep. A lightweight blanket should be used so she doesn't get too hot. And once your baby is able to turn over from back to front or able to escape from the blanket, you should stop swaddling her at sleep time. Loose blankets in a crib can increase the risk of sudden infant death syndrome (SIDS).

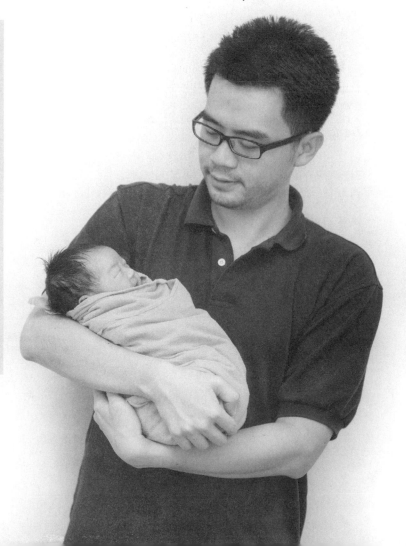

Maria's Story

Isabel cried an awful lot when we first got home. It seemed like I could never put her down. I was so tired. All I wanted to do was sleep. I'd walk with her, rock her, and try to sing to her and play with her all the time, but it wore me out. Finally, someone told me to try swaddling her. I used this stretchy baby blanket to wrap her up like a little burrito. She calmed down, especially when I said, "Shhhh," over and over again. It really helped. I swaddled her a lot in those first 3 months. Someone else recommended that I buy a sling or baby carrier, and that really helped too. I was able to carry her like she wanted me to, and still have my hands free to get other things done. The leader of the mother-baby group talked about how we can overstimulate our babies if we do too much, so I make sure we have some quiet times every day where she's just hanging out and looking around.

Supplies for Baby Care

What do you need for your newborn baby? There's very little that's really required. Here are a few basics:

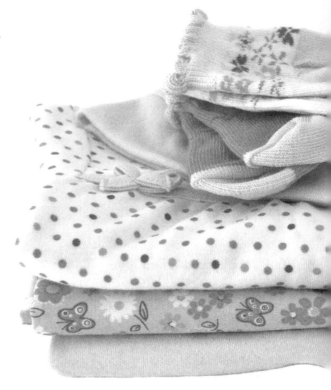

Bed

- crib, *bassinet* (baby bed), *cosleeper* (bassinet that attaches to your bed), or have your baby in your bed
- 2–3 sheets for crib or bed
- waterproof mattress pad
- 3–6 large, lightweight cotton baby blankets
- 1–2 blanket sleepers (footie pajamas) or sleep sacks

Bath

- 1–2 soft towels
- 2–3 washcloths
- baby soap and shampoo
- cotton swabs for umbilical cord
- baby bathtub if desired

Diapers

- 4 dozen cloth diapers (or diaper service) plus 5–6 waterproof wraps OR 70 disposable diapers per week
- 6–8 thin washcloths or a box of diaper wipes
- changing table (you could also use a table or counter with a folded towel for padding)

Baby clothes

- 4–6 undershirts or "onesies"
- 4–6 outfits and/or gowns
- 2–4 pairs of socks or booties
- hat and warm sweater or jacket during the cold months

Travel

- car seat
- diaper bag (or large purse or tote bag)

Other equipment (if desired)

- digital thermometer
- front pack or sling to help you hold your baby
- stroller
- large exercise ball for bouncing your baby
- baby swing

How to Comfort Your Crying Baby

Watching for cues can give you some ideas about what your baby might need. Sometimes if you meet her needs right away, she won't cry. But other times, no matter what you do, she will cry. You may get upset when your baby cries. This is a natural reaction. Remind yourself that your first job is to meet her needs; then if she's still crying, your job is to hold her and soothe her. Your job is not to make her stop crying—that could be impossible. Remind yourself when she's crying that it doesn't mean you're a bad parent! When she begins crying, respond quickly before she gets so upset that you can't calm her easily. Start by making sure her basic needs are met:

- *Feed your baby.* It might seem to you like a short time since she last ate, but it might seem like a long time to her. If she's not interested in eating, try letting her suck on your finger or a pacifier.
- If she seems gassy or needs to burp, try holding her in a position that puts pressure on her tummy (see page 136).
- Make sure your baby isn't too warm or too cold. Also, check to see if she needs a diaper change.
- Swaddle her.

Once you've made sure that her needs are met, then don't worry more about *why* she's crying. Just accept it, and focus on soothing her. Choose one of these soothing methods and use it for a while. Try not to overstimulate her by quickly changing from 1 method to another.

- Hold her on your arm with her facing away from you. Gently sway back and forth to comfort her.
- Walk around with her in a front pack or sling.
- Hold her in your arms as you gently bounce for several minutes. Try bouncing while standing or while sitting on a bed or exercise ball.
- Sit in a rocking chair and rock back and forth.
- Take her outside for a stroller ride. A car ride also may help your baby fall asleep.
- Put her in a baby swing for a while. Make sure her head is supported as she gently swings.
- Sing a quiet song to her. (It doesn't have to be a lullaby. If all you can remember at the moment is the theme song of a TV show or an ad jingle, it's fine to sing that.)
- While cuddling or rocking her, try using white noise. (This reminds babies of the sounds they heard in the womb.) Some parents make "shhhh" sounds near their baby's ear. Some run the bathroom fan, the clothes dryer, or a vacuum.
- Try the 5 S's method by Harvey Karp. Search for it on YouTube, or check out his book or DVD *The Happiest Baby on the Block*. It combines many of the ideas above into a standard routine.

Try something for five minutes. If she continues to cry after five minutes, try something else. You'll find a method that works. With time and practice, you'll become better at comforting your baby.

Some parents worry that if they give their baby too much attention, they'll spoil her. A newborn baby can't be spoiled. She can't take care of herself. She needs you to do everything for her (feeding, dressing, bathing, and comforting). Taking care of your baby's needs is not spoiling her.

When your baby cries, she needs *more* care, not less. And the sooner you pick up a crying baby, the sooner the crying stops. By responding to her cries, you're showing her that you're listening to her. And when her needs are met, over time she'll cry less.

Cami's Story

Some of my friends told me a few tricks to help Tommy calm down from crying or get him to sleep. One told me that when her little boy couldn't settle down, she put him in the stroller and walked outside. She even went out when it was raining because her stroller had a rain cover. Another friend danced with her baby with the music up pretty loud. As her baby started to calm down, she slowed down and turned the music down too. Another friend told Chris to hold the baby and sit on a big exercise ball and bounce gently up and down. Tommy loved that!

What If Your Baby Cries a Lot?

All new babies have fussy times. Often these times occur in the evening. As your baby grows older, this newborn fussiness will end. Many babies experience something called "the period of PURPLE crying" between 2 weeks and 3 months. To know if your baby is experiencing this, follow these clues:

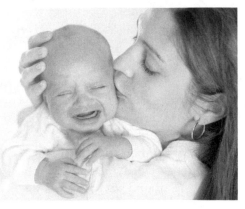

- P (peak of crying): Your baby cries more each week, the most around 2 months. Then he starts crying less each week.
- U (unexpected): Crying comes and goes, and you can't figure out why.
- R (resists soothing): You try all the calming techniques above, and your baby still cries.
- P (painful expression): Your baby looks like he's in pain, though he's not.
- L (long-lasting): Your baby cries for several hours a day.
- E (evening): Most babies cry more in the evening.

(See www.purplecrying.info to learn more.)

When your baby is in this period of PURPLE crying, remind yourself that it's not your fault, and that you may not always be able to stop him from crying. You may just need to hold him while he cries. Try to find some way to take care of yourself and keep yourself calm during this time (go for a walk, listen to music on headphones).

Have a plan for what you'll do when things get really hard. If nothing seems to calm your baby and you're losing your temper, take a short break. If you have help at home, let someone else try to comfort him. If not, put your baby down safely in his crib or car seat for 5–10 minutes and move at least 10 feet away while you calm down. Never shake or hurt your baby. Don't treat him roughly. Call someone (a friend or relative) to help you. Tell the person you need a break.

If you think your baby cries a lot more than other babies, talk with his doctor. The doctor may encourage you to take him in for a checkup or may suggest other ways to cope with the crying.

Maria's Story

The mother-baby class saved my life. I found out there are other babies just like Isabel. And other mothers are stressed out too. The group leader talked about "high-needs" babies. That's definitely Isabel. Our leader told us that these babies settle down after a while. She told us not to think that our babies don't like us or that we're terrible mothers. I needed to hear that. Our leader also said that being home alone all day with a baby is hard. Some of the mothers in the group made plans to meet at the park once a week. It was nice to have adults around who understood what I was going through. I looked forward to our classes and going to the park.

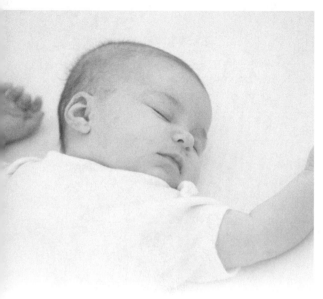

Your Baby's Sleep

Watch your baby for tired cues. First, he may just get a blank expression and not really want to connect with you. Then he may begin to yawn, or rub his eyes (or his nose or his forehead—babies aren't always good at rubbing their eyes), or turn his head side to side, as if trying to find a comfortable spot. You can begin to soothe him to sleep.

Any of the techniques we described for soothing a baby from crying to calm also work to soothe a baby from calm to sleep. You just do them at a different "volume level." For example, if you had a baby crying very loudly, you might bounce up and down with a lot of energy and sing a lullaby loudly so the baby can hear you. If you have a sleepy baby, you would bounce or sway gently and sing quietly.

Babies often fall asleep while nursing. So change your baby's diaper *before* you nurse. Then, when she's almost done eating and starting to fall asleep, gently lay the baby down. (*Tip*: if you set an almost-asleep baby in the crib on her back, she will often startle awake. Instead, hold her on her side as you lower her down into the crib, then gently roll her onto her back, and rub her arm or belly for a few minutes till she falls asleep.)

Sleep Patterns

A newborn baby sleeps between 12 and 20 hours each day. But he usually sleeps for only a short time and then wakes up to eat. (In the diagram, the dark portions show when a baby might be sleeping during a 24 hour day, and the light areas show when the baby is awake.) Remember, most newborn babies nurse 10 or more times each day.

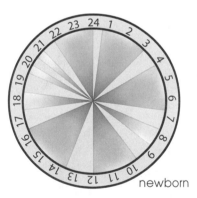

newborn

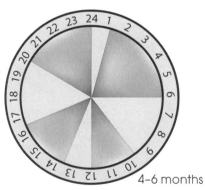

4–6 months

Many babies have a few longer periods of sleep (3–4 hours) every day. They have other periods of the day when they're more awake and want to feed every 1–2 hours. These "cluster feeds" often happen in the evening.

At first, your baby's schedule will seem new and different each day. As your baby gets older, you may be able to get your baby on a sleep schedule, but it's very hard with a baby younger than 3 months. Newborns don't really know day from night and are just as likely to be awake to feed at 2:00 AM as they are at 2:00 PM. You can help them learn the difference. In the daytime, turn on the lights and make noise, even during naptime. At night, keep things quiet and dark.

These sleep patterns are normal and healthy for a newborn. However, these sleep patterns may be hard for parents to handle! Check out our tips for coping with sleep issues on page 123.

Sleep Location

Having your baby sleep in your room (in a crib or bassinet) instead of in a different room reduces the risk of sudden infant death syndrome (SIDS). Babies who sleep in the same room as their parents may wake up more often at night, but the wakeups are usually quieter. The parents are often able to meet the baby's needs before she starts crying. A baby who sleeps in a different room may be crying hard by the time her parents get to her. They have to calm her before they can meet her needs and soothe her back to sleep. This can lead to less total sleep for the parents.

Many parents plan to sleep with their babies in their beds, perhaps because it's common in their culture. Other parents who never planned to bed-share do it because they find it's the only way to manage nighttime challenges. The American Academy of Pediatrics (AAP) recommends room-sharing, but discourages bed-sharing.

If you do choose to bed-share, it's important that you follow the safer sleep practices detailed in the section below. Learn more about safer bed-sharing practices at http://cosleeping.nd.edu.

> ### Warning
>
> If you or your partner smoke, drink alcohol, use drugs, or take medicines that make you sleepy, or if either of you are obese, your baby should not sleep in the same bed with you. You could roll onto your baby without knowing it.

Sudden Infant Death Syndrome (SIDS)

Many parents worry about SIDS, the unexpected death of a healthy baby. About 1 in 2,000 babies dies of SIDS. It usually occurs while a baby is asleep or in bed and is most common between 2 and 4 months of age. SIDS is not caused by suffocation, spitting up, vaccines, or child abuse. Here's what you can do to reduce your baby's risk:

- Keep your baby away from tobacco smoke and from people and clothing that smell of smoke. This is important during pregnancy and after he's born.
- Breastfeed. Breastfeeding lowers the risk of SIDS.
- No matter where your baby sleeps, follow these safer sleep practices:
  - Always place your baby on his back on a firm surface. Make sure that anyone caring for your baby places him on his back to sleep.
  - Keep your baby warm but not hot. Dress him in the same amount of clothing as you're wearing plus a lightweight blanket sleeper that substitutes for a blanket.
  - Remove soft toys, pillows, lambskins, and comforters from his sleeping area.
  - See page 159 about swaddling safely.

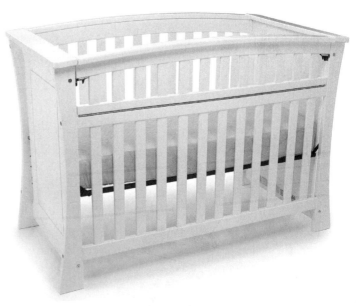

Keeping Your Baby Healthy and Safe

You can help protect your new baby from getting sick by washing your hands often while you care for her. It gets rid of most germs. Also, ask your friends and family members to wash their hands before holding or touching your baby.

Health Care for Your Baby

Right after birth, the medical staff at the hospital will check your baby. Your baby's doctor may also examine her at the hospital before you go home.

The hospital staff performs tests to see if your baby is healthy, including a hearing test, a test for heart defects, and a blood test to screen for inherited diseases. (You can find out the tests done in your state by going to the March of Dimes website at www.marchofdimes.com.)

If you have a baby boy, you'll be asked about *circumcision* (removal of the skin at the end of the penis). If you choose to have him circumcised, it may be done before he leaves the hospital. Or your doctor or your baby's doctor may do the procedure at a clinic during the first week after birth. There are different medical benefits and risks for circumcising and for not circumcising, so there's not a clear medical reason to do it or not to do it. It is a personal and religious choice. Circumcision isn't usually covered by insurance, so you'll probably have to pay for it yourself. Not as many boys are circumcised now as they were in the past. Talk to your baby's doctor about your decision on circumcision.

Most families choose their baby's health-care provider before birth. This may be a pediatrician, a family doctor, or a clinic with doctors and nurse practitioners. The person you choose depends on where you live and the kind of care you want. Your choice also depends on the type of health-care coverage you have. If you don't have medical insurance, talk to your caregiver or clinic nurse to find out how to get free or low-cost medical care. Or call the Insure Kids Now! hotline at 877-KIDS-NOW (877-543-7669).

It's nice to talk to your baby's health-care provider before the birth. You can talk about your choices for newborn care in the hospital. You can also plan your baby's first visit after the birth. Your baby needs to have a checkup when he's 3–10 days old. He'll be weighed to see if he's getting enough to eat. He'll also be checked for *jaundice* (yellow skin color that comes from too much bilirubin in the blood).

During his first year, your baby will be seen on a regular schedule to check on his growth and health. Your baby's health-care provider will let you know when you'll need to make appointments. In the days before each visit, write down questions you think of and bring the list to the appointment to remind you of your questions.

Tanya's Story

After Michael was born, my best friend wanted to come see him and bring her little girl, Lauren, to play with Molly. As we talked, she told me that Lauren missed school all week with a cold and sore throat. I got nervous because I didn't want Michael or Molly to catch something. My friend said Lauren wasn't spreading germs anymore. But I told her I wanted to wait a few days. Maybe I was being overprotective, but I didn't want my kids getting sick. I was still tired, and Michael was so young.

Immunizations

Your baby needs *immunizations* (shots or *vaccines*) to protect her from serious infections. Although most of these diseases are rare in the United States, these germs are still around and can cause serious problems for your baby. Having immunizations will protect your baby and people around her. You'll also need a record of your child's shots when you take her to child care or preschool.

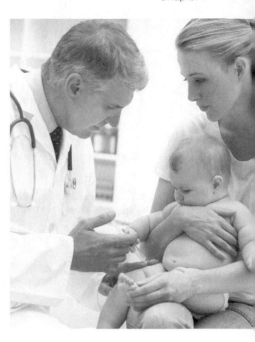

Immunization shots are given at several times during your baby's first years. Then *booster shots* (repeat doses) are given at specific ages as your child grows older. Vaccines are often mixed together in 1 shot so fewer shots are needed at each visit. Your baby's health-care provider will tell you when shots are needed for your baby.

Immunizations Are Important

Vaccine shots keep your baby healthy. They help prevent diseases that could seriously harm you or your baby.

There are some side effects to immunizations. The common effects are mild and only last a day or two. Many babies are fussy for a few hours or days after a vaccine shot. It's normal for the injection site to be sore and tender. Some babies have a low fever.

Make sure to tell your health-care provider if your baby has a more serious reaction, such as a high fever, severe rash, *seizure* (convulsion), or crying that lasts more than 3 hours. If you can't reach your doctor or clinic, take your baby to an urgent care clinic or the emergency room. These serious reactions are rare, but they might be harmful.

Although you may worry that immunizing your baby will increase the risk of autism, you shouldn't. Research hasn't shown a link between the two. There is a lot of wrong information about vaccines on the Internet, so be sure you're looking at good information. One source is: http://here.doh.wa.gov /materials/plaintalk.

Taking Your Baby's Temperature

To quickly find out if your baby might have a fever, put your hand on your baby's chest. Then touch the back of your neck. If your baby's chest feels hotter than your neck, check his temperature.

You can take your baby's temperature by putting a digital thermometer under his arm (*axillary* temperature). Do not put a thermometer in your baby's mouth (oral temperature) until he is older than 5 years. It helps to know that a normal body temperature is different depending on the area of the body used.

- A normal underarm temperature is about 97.6°F.
- A normal rectal temperature is about 99.6°F.
- A normal oral temperature is about 98.6°F.

How to Use Your Thermometer

Turn on the thermometer. When it's ready, put it in your baby's armpit. Bring her arm down and hold it against her body. Wait until the digital thermometer beeps and then read it. Clean the thermometer by washing the tip with soap and warm water. Or you can you wipe it with a cotton ball that's been dipped in rubbing alcohol.

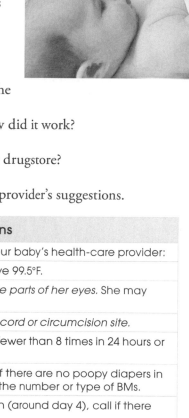

When to Call for Medical Help

If you're worried about your baby's health, call his doctor or health clinic. You can call whenever you have questions. You don't have to wait until your baby is seriously sick.

When you call, here are some things the doctor or nurse may ask:

- What's your baby's temperature? (Take it before you call.)
- What symptoms do you notice? Is your baby coughing? Is he vomiting? Is there a rash?
- Is your baby fussier than usual? Is he acting differently from the way he usually acts? Is he very sleepy or floppy when awake?
- Is your baby eating normally? Are his bowel movements the same as usual?
- What have you done to treat the illness or condition? How did it work?
- Is anyone else sick at home or child care?
- What's the name and phone number of your pharmacy or drugstore?

Have a paper and pencil handy to write down the health-care provider's suggestions.

Newborn Warning Signs
If you notice any of these signs in the first month, call your baby's health-care provider:
Fever. Call if your baby's underarm temperature is above 99.5°F.
Yellowish color to your baby's face, chest, and the white parts of her eyes. She may have jaundice.
Bright red bleeding or foul-smelling pus appears at the cord or circumcision site.
Problems with feeding. Call if your newborn baby eats fewer than 8 times in 24 hours or has trouble waking up for feedings.
Problems with bowel movements. In the first week, call if there are no poopy diapers in a 24-hour period. Later, call if there are big changes in the number or type of BMs.
Not enough wet diapers. After your breast milk comes in (around day 4), call if there are fewer than 6 wet diapers in a 24-hour day.
Problems with breathing. Call 911 if your baby has blue lips or is struggling to breathe.
Call if anything about your baby causes you to be worried or concerned.

Car Safety

Babies and children need to be in car seats when riding in a car. It's the law in the United States. A car seat can save your baby's life if it's put in correctly and used every time your baby rides in the car.

Here are some suggestions:

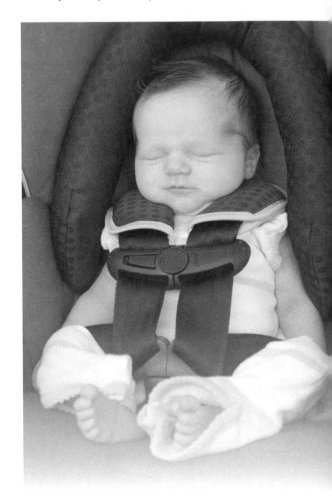

- Use the right size and type of car seat. Babies are placed in rear-facing car seats until they are at least 2 years old.
- If you don't have the money to buy a car seat, ask your caregiver or social worker how to get a low-cost or free one.
- Before the baby is born, properly fasten the seat into your car. Read the directions for both the car seat and the car you'll be using. Sometimes it's hard to get it in just right. Some hospitals and other agencies offer free car seat safety checks to make sure you've installed your car seat correctly. To find a car seat check near you, go to http://www.seatcheck.org.
- Put the car seat in the back seat, ideally in the middle of the back seat. Keep your baby away from air bags.
- The car seat harness should be snug over your baby's shoulders. The harness clip should be at the same level as your baby's armpits.
- Avoid dressing your baby in a bulky coat or wrapping your baby in blankets. Put him in the car seat in regular clothes and then put a blanket over him.
- Be careful about adding car seat pads. These can make your car seat unsafe. Instead, use a rolled-up towel or small blanket tucked in around your baby's head for support.

To learn more about car seats, go to http://www.safercar.gov/parents.

Safety at Home

In the first few months after birth, here are some ways to protect your baby:

* Keep your baby away from *secondhand smoke* (smoke from a cigarette or cigar). Babies who are exposed to secondhand smoke have more colds and ear infections. And they're at increased risk of sudden infant death syndrome (SIDS).
* Have a safe place for your baby to sleep (see page 164).
* Keep at least 1 hand on your baby when she's on a changing table, bed, or other high surface that she could fall off of.
* Watch your baby when young children are around. Most little kids don't know what's dangerous for a new baby. A toddler might think he's helping you by picking up your baby when she's crying. A child older than 10 years usually knows what's safe.
* Don't play roughly with your baby. Be gentle. Never throw her up in the air. And never shake her.
* Babies need good head support in the first months. Even when your baby can hold her head up well, she still needs to be handled gently.
* Don't have strings or cords near your baby. She could wrap them around her neck and choke. Avoid strings on her clothing, near her crib, and attached to her pacifier.

As your baby grows and becomes more active, she needs your help to stay safe. Babies who crawl and climb are more likely to get hurt. When your baby is about 4–6 months old, you should start baby-proofing your home.

For more information on child safety, see the safety resources listed in the back of the book.

Cami's Story

Don't learn about baby safety the hard way, like I did. I thought Tommy couldn't roll over. He was only 3 months old. I left him on the bed while I went to the bathroom. I had just finishing washing my hands when I heard a CLUNK! I ran into the room. There he was on the floor beside the bed. He must have worked his way off the bed while I was in the bathroom. Luckily, he was okay. I felt so guilty. Now I know that I need to do things to keep him safe, even if I think he can't get himself into any trouble yet.

Your Baby's Growth and Development

Your baby will change so much over the first two years of life. To help your baby's brain grow, she needs three things:

- *Novelty*. Your baby loves new experiences. And almost everything is new to a baby! See ideas below for ways to play with your baby.
- *Repetition*. Your baby likes to do the same thing over and over to help her learn. She also likes routines—knowing that you'll respond to her the same way every time helps her learn about her world.
- *Rest*. Your baby also needs some quiet time to absorb and process all this information. Have some quiet times each day. Turn off the TV and the music, put away the busy baby toys, and let your child just quietly gaze around her.

There are lots of skills your baby will develop: social, language, problem-solving, and motor skills (knowing how to use her body). It's helpful for you to know about normal developmental milestones and how to know if she's able to do the things she should be able to. Subscribe to *Just in Time Parenting*, a free e-mail newsletter about development at http://jitp.extension.org. Or look at the website for Zero to Three to learn about development and how you can help: http://www.zerotothree.org.

Playing with Your Baby

It's fun to play with your baby. Also, play is the way your baby learns about himself and the world around him. At first, although he can't do much, you can sing to your baby or dance with him. He may enjoy being stroked or having a massage. You can show him things, and talk to him about what you're doing. Let him smell things like food, flowers, and candies. Enjoy playing in the bathtub together. Take him outdoors in all different weather and seasons. Playing games such as peekaboo will be fun for both of you. When your baby gets a little older, he'll enjoy rattles, books, and simple toys. He will be just as happy to play with a spoon and a pot as with an expensive toy from the store. (For ideas on how to play with your child from age 1–5, see www.gooddays withkids.com.)

Play with your baby when he's awake, alert, and calm. Give him a break when he starts to zone out. (See information about playtime and break-time cues on page 154.)

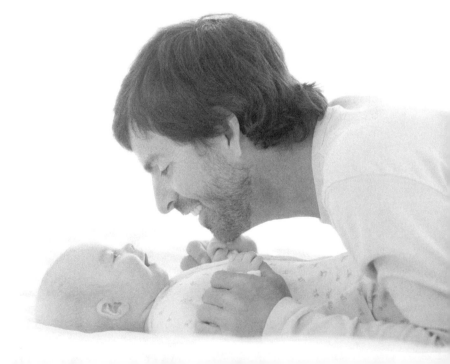

Tummy Time

Between time spent in the car seat and bouncer seats and always sleeping on her back, a baby can develop a flat spot on the back of her head. When your baby is awake, let her spend time in different positions. Here are some ways to give her time off her back to help her neck and back muscles become stronger:

- Put her on her tummy on a firm surface that allows her to lift her head. If she gets fussy, place some safe toys in front of her to look at, or lie down next to her.
- Hold your baby in your arms, a sling, or a front pack.

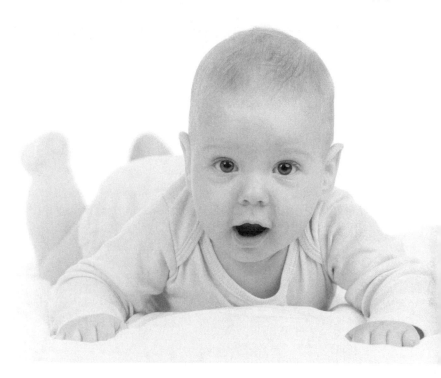

Note to Fathers and Partners

When your baby first comes home, it may seem like the baby's mother is better at taking care of the baby than you are. You'll be surprised at how much fathers and partners can do:

- If your baby is breastfed, help feed your baby by making sure your baby's mother eats well every day. This helps her make breast milk for your baby. When she's nursing, bring her pillows or water or keep her company.
- If your baby is bottle-fed, help with feeding and with washing bottles.
- Become the diaper changing expert of the family.
- Bathe the baby. This can be a special time for you and your baby. You might try taking your baby into the tub or shower with you. Be careful, though, as babies are slippery when wet.
- Relax while your baby takes a nap with you. Lean back with your baby lying on your chest. You'll both love it.
- Dance or walk with your baby. Sway to the music. Sing to him. He knows your voice and feels safe in your arms.
- Rock in a rocking chair or gently bounce on a big exercise ball. Babies love movement.
- Take your baby for a stroller ride. Getting out of the house can be good for the whole family.
- Take on the responsibility of scheduling your baby's well-child checkups, and go along on doctor visits.

You're an important part of your child's life. By being with your baby in the first weeks and months, you'll get to know each other. You'll be amazed at how deeply and quickly you fall in love with your new baby.

A Note to Families Having Another Baby

Older children may or may not be excited about having a new baby. Even if they're excited before the baby comes, that can change once the baby is in your home night and day. One thing is certain: life is never the same for the older child (or for you) after the birth of a new baby.

Your older child's behavior may surprise and disappoint you during the first weeks after your baby's birth. Your child may react in a variety of ways:

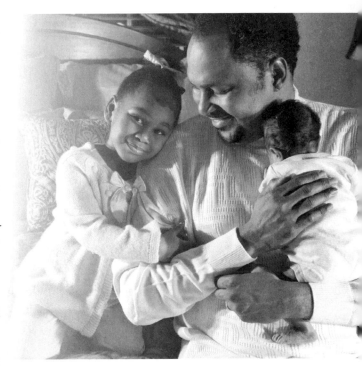

- She may go back to wanting to breastfeed or take a bottle, sucking her thumb, or wetting her pants.
- She may throw temper tantrums.
- She may be angry with you or the baby.
- She may not pay attention to the baby, or she may ignore you.
- Her sleeping and eating habits may change.
- She may be nice and helpful with the baby.

What can you do to help your older child adjust?
- Prepare your child before the baby's born. Tell her about babies. Read books about being an older brother or sister. Talk with her and find out what she knows about babies and being an older sibling.
- Try to accept your child's reactions as normal responses to stress. Don't let your child harm herself or the baby, but understand her feelings.
- Plan some time alone with your older child.
- Show her photos of you caring for her as a baby.
- Let her help you with baby care if she wants. Be sure to stay with your children when they're together.
- When visitors bring gifts for the baby, let your older child open them. You may encourage visitors to bring a gift for your older child too.

Tanya's Story

Taking care of our baby was so much easier the second time. I knew how to change diapers, give him a bath, and soothe him when he cried. So I didn't worry as much. After a while, Molly started paying attention to Michael. She sang and danced for him. She even nursed her doll while I was breastfeeding. That was fun to see. I was glad when she started enjoying her baby brother. It felt like we were finally becoming a family!

Help for You and Your Baby

This list provides information about organizations and services that might be helpful during pregnancy and after having your baby. You can also ask your doctor, midwife, or childbirth educator for local resources.

We also encourage you to look at http://www.pcnguide.com. It is the companion website for our other book *Pregnancy, Childbirth, and the Newborn* and includes lots more resources on all of these topics.

Preconception Resources

Fertility Help:
Centers for Disease Control on Assisted Reproductive Technology (ART)
www.cdc.gov/art/index.html
800-CDC-INFO
This agency has information on using medical fertility treatments to get pregnant.

Fertility Friend
www.fertilityfriend.com
This website will help you pinpoint when you're ovulating and most likely to get pregnant.

General Pregnancy and Birth Resources

Having a Healthy Pregnancy:
Office on Women's Health
www.womenshealth.gov/pregnancy/index.html
This website provides a pregnancy overview with links to other great resources.

March of Dimes
www.marchofdimes.org
This group provides information and support about having a safe pregnancy and healthy baby, with an emphasis on preventing preterm birth.

US Department of Agriculture's My Plate
www.choosemyplate.gov
This website will help you figure out how much of each food group is right for you to eat while pregnant and breastfeeding.

Lamaze International's "Your Pregnancy Week by Week"
www.lamaze.org
Lamaze International's free weekly e-mail newsletter features information, tips, and stories to help guide women and families through pregnancy and beyond.

The National Healthy Mothers, Healthy Babies Coalition (HMHB)'s "Text4baby"
www.text4baby.org
This free (in the United States) text messaging service provides accurate, text-length information about your pregnancy.

Making Informed Choices about Pregnancy and Birth:
Childbirth Connection
www.childbirthconnection.org
Childbirth Connection works to improve the quality of maternity care and provides information to help women make the right choices for their care.

Mother's Advocate
www.mothersadvocate.org
This website offers free video clips to help women learn about choices they can make or maternity practices they can ask for to have a safe and healthy birth.

Resources to Help You Avoid Hazards

Smoking:
Centers for Disease Control Tobacco Information and Prevention Source (TIPS)
www.cdc.gov/tobacco/quit_smoking/cessation/index.htm
800-CDC-INFO
Their website offers resources to help you stop smoking.

Alcohol:
Alcoholics Anonymous (AA)
www.aa.org
Search this organization's website for resources to help you stop drinking alcohol.

Drugs:
Narcotics Anonymous (NA)
www.na.org
This organization offers resources to help you stop drug use.

Substance Abuse and Mental Health Services Administration (SAMHSA)
www.samhsa.gov
800-662-HELP (800-662-4357)
This agency has support centers around the United States to help people who need treatment.

Domestic Violence:
The National Domestic Violence Hotline (NDVH)
www.ndvh.org
800-799-SAFE (800-799-7233)
This organization helps victims of abuse and violence. Contact them if you need suggestions on how to handle a bad relationship.

Workplace Hazards:
Centers for Disease Control National Institute for Occupational Safety and Health (NIOSH)
www.cdc.gov/niosh/topics/repro
800-CDC-INFO
This agency has information on how to prevent workplace exposures to hazards.

Medications and All Other Hazards:
Organization of Teratology Specialists (OTIS)
www.mothertobaby.org
866-626-6847
This organization provides information for parents and health-care professionals about possible hazards for babies during pregnancy and breastfeeding.

Resources for Choosing Caregivers

Find an Obstetrician (Ob-Gyn):
American Congress of Obstetricians and Gynecologists (ACOG)
www.acog.org
This organization has the names of obstetricians in your state. Also, most hospitals have a list of doctors who deliver babies there.

Find a Family Practice Doctor or Other Caregiver Who Delivers at Your Preferred Hospital:
Check your hospital's website for a list of caregivers who deliver babies there.

Find a Certified Nurse-Midwife (CNM):
American College of Nurse-Midwives (ACNM)
www.midwife.org/find-a-midwife
240-485-1800
This organization can help you find one in your area.

Find a Licensed Midwife (LM):
Mothers Naturally
http://mothersnaturally.org/midwives/findAMidwife.php
Go to this website and enter your city and state to find a midwife near you.

Citizens for Midwifery
http://cfmidwifery.org/find
This website contains information about what midwives do and also has several directories to help you find one in your area.

Find a Birth Center:
American Association of Childbearing Centers
www.birthcenters.org/search/custom.asp?id=2926
This association can help you find one in your area.

Low-Cost Care Resources

Information about Local Public Health Clinics:
US Department of Health and Human Services Hotline
800-311-BABY (800-311-2229)
This toll-free hotline can connect you to your local health department.

Medicaid Information:
Medicaid.gov
www.medicaid.gov
This website has information about Medicaid funds for pregnant women and children younger than 6 years old whose family income is less than a certain amount. You can apply for Medicaid and for the Children's Health Insurance Program (CHIP) at http://www.healthcare.gov.

For Help Getting Food:
Women, Infants, and Children (WIC)
www.fns.usda.gov/wic
The WIC program offers food for pregnant women and breastfeeding help for new mothers whose income is less than a certain amount. They can help you find parenting assistance and support. Also, your caregiver may help you find your local WIC office.

National Hunger Hotline
866-3-HUNGRY (866-348-6479)
This hotline will connect you to government assistance programs and information on emergency food distribution.

Childbirth Classes and Birth Partner Resources

Find a Doula:
Doulas of North America (DONA)
www.dona.org
888-788-DONA (888-788-3662)
This organization can help you find a doula (a professional birth partner) in your area.

Doula Match
www.doulamatch.net
This website will help match you with a birth or postpartum doula.

Find Childbirth Educators and Classes:
International Childbirth Education Association (ICEA)
www.icea.org
800-624-4934
This association provides information about finding a childbirth educator in your area.

Lamaze International
www.lamaze.org
This organization provides information about how to find a Lamaze childbirth class near you.

Your Local Hospital
Contact your local hospital to see if it offers classes.

Baby Care Resources

Raising a healthy child:
American Academy of Pediatrics (AAP)
www.healthychildren.org
This organization offers information about keeping your child healthy, parenting, and finding a pediatrician (doctor for babies and children).

Seattle Children's Hospital
www.seattlechildrens.org/safety-wellness
This website features videos and articles about injury prevention, nutrition, and other topics to keep your child healthy and safe.

Home Safety and Unsafe Product Recalls:
Consumer Product Safety Commission (CPSC)
www.cpsc.gov
800-638-2772
This agency offers information about home safety and unsafe baby care products.

Immunization Information:
Immunization Action Coalition
www.immunize.org
651-647-9009
This organization offers information about shots to keep your baby healthy.

National Immunization Hotline
800-232-2522
This hotline will give you answers to any questions you may have about shots.

Car Seat Information:
National Highway Traffic Safety Administration (NHTSA)
www.nhtsa.gov/Safety/CPS
Their Parents Central department offers information about infant and child car seats.

Information about Safe Sleeping and Sudden Infant Death Syndrome (SIDS):
First Candle
www.sidsalliance.org
800-221-7437
This organization provides information about SIDS and other causes of infant death. They offer suggestions about safe sleeping.

American SIDS Institute
http://sids.org/what-is-sidssuid/reduce-the-risk
239-431-5425
This group offers education about prevention and counseling for families who have lost a child to SIDS.

Breastfeeding Resources

Find a Lactation Consultant:
International Lactation Consultant Association (ILCA)
www.ilca.org
919-861-5577
This association keeps records of breastfeeding professionals who are International Board Certified Lactation Consultants (IBCLCs). Contact them to find a breastfeeding expert in your area.

Breastfeeding Support:
La Leche League (LLL)
www.llli.org
800-LALECHE (800-525-3243)
This organization offers mother-baby groups for breastfeeding support. Contact them to find a LLL group near you. Or ask them to help you find breastfeeding consultants in your area.

Office on Women's Health
www.womenshealth.gov/breastfeeding/index.html
800-994-9662
This agency answers breastfeeding questions. Their website has helpful information and links to other resources.

Parenting Resources

General Parenting Help:
Healthy Mothers, Healthy Babies Coalition (HMHB)
www.hmhb.org/family.html
703-837-4792
This organization offers help with breastfeeding and parenting.

Your Local Community College
Check to see if it has parenting classes.

Information for Fathers:
Great Dads
www.greatdads.com
This website offers parenting tips and information from a father's perspective.

Information about Colic or Excessive Crying:
Period of Purple Crying
www.purplecrying.info
This website helps parents understand colic and gives tips on dealing with a baby who won't stop crying.

Information for Parents of Multiples:
Multiples of America
www.multiplesofamerica.org/
This organization provides information and support for women having more than 1 baby. Contact them to learn the names of local groups for parents of multiples.

Information about Child Development:
Parenting Counts
www.parentingcounts.org
The program offers information focused on the social and emotional development of babies and young children.

Zero to Three
www.zerotothree.org/parenting-resources
This nonprofit has many resources for parents who want to know more about their child's development, including a series of podcasts called *Little Kids, Big Questions*.

Find Support for Single Parents:
Parents Without Partners
www.parentswithoutpartners.org
800-637-7974
This organization provides information and support for single parents and their children. Contact them to find a group in your area.

Information on Birth Control and Family Planning:
Planned Parenthood
www.plannedparenthood.org
800-230-PLAN (800-230-7526)
This organization can tell you about methods you can use to avoid getting pregnant.

Postpartum Depression and Loss Resources

For Help with a Perinatal Mood Disorder:
Postpartum Support International
www.postpartum.net
800-944-4PPD (800-944-4773)
This group offers help to women with a perinatal mood disorder, such as postpartum depression. Contact them to learn about a mothers' support group in your area.

For Help with Loss:
Share Pregnancy & Infant Loss Support:
www.nationalshare.org
800-821-6819
This group offers support for families who have lost a baby by early pregnancy loss, stillbirth, or newborn death.

Glossary

The following are terms that are used to describe
pregnancy, childbirth, and newborn care.

4-1-1 or 5-1-1 rule
This rule means that your labor contractions are intense enough to require you to focus and breathe rhythmically through them, and are *four
or five* minutes apart with each lasting at least *one minute* for a period of
one hour. This pattern signals to you that your labor may be progressing
and it's time to call your caregiver or birthplace.

abnormal fetal heart rate
Term used when your baby's heart rate isn't responding to contractions
in a reassuring way. Doesn't necessarily indicate that something is wrong
with your baby (there's a high rate of "false positives"); however, it does
indicate the need for closer monitoring and a possible need for intervention in labor.

active labor
The second phase of the first stage of labor. When your cervix is dilated
to 4 to 5 centimeters, your contractions usually reach the 4-1-1 or 5-1-1
pattern. During this phase, dilation usually speeds up, contractions typically become painful (but manageable), and labor progresses with each
contraction.

acupuncture
An ancient Chinese medicine technique that uses needles placed at
strategic points along meridians, or energy flow lines, in your body to
guide it toward wellness and balance.

advanced practice nurse practitioner
A maternity caregiver who provides prenatal and postpartum care, but
doesn't attend women during labor.

afterpains
As your uterus contracts after birth to its nonpregnant size (a process
called involution), you may experience periods of discomfort or pain.
Although this pain is common and isn't nearly as intense as labor
contractions, you may need to use slow breathing to help manage it in the
first few days.

alveoli
Glands in the breast that produce and store milk.

amniocentesis
A medical procedure in which a needle is used to withdraw a small
amount of amniotic fluid from your uterus. A laboratory analyzes the
surfactant levels in the fluid to determine whether your baby's lungs are
mature enough to function outside your womb.

amnioinfusion
A procedure in which fluids are infused into your uterus to dilute any
meconium that was expelled in the amniotic fluid , or to remove pressure
on the cord caused by your baby's head or trunk.

amniotic fluid
The fluid that surrounds your baby in the amniotic sac. It protects
your baby by absorbing bumps from the outside, maintaining an
even temperature, providing a medium for easy movement, and
allowing your baby to develop her lungs by "breathing" the fluid.

amniotic sac
Made up of the membranes (amnion and chorion) that create the sac
that surrounds your baby. Also called "bag of waters."

amniotomy
See *artificial rupture of membranes (AROM)*.

analgesia
Any effect that reduces your perception of pain. In this book, this term
is used to refer specifically to medications that act on the brain so you
don't recognize pain stimuli or don't interpret them as pain.

androgens
Male hormones that signal the development of a baby boy's scrotum
and penis.

anemia
A condition in which the number of red blood cells is lower than
normal, reducing the blood's capacity to carry oxygen.

anesthesia
Indicates a loss of sensation, including pain sensation. Anesthetic medications block nerve endings from sending pain impulses to your brain.

antibodies
Proteins that protect your body from bacteria and toxins. During pregnancy and breastfeeding, your baby receives antibodies from you, which
will protect him against diseases to which you're resistant or immune.

Apgar score
Within one minute after your baby's birth and again at five
minutes, your caregiver will evaluate your baby's well-being by
conducting this routine newborn assessment, which assesses
how well she's adapting to life outside your womb.

areola
The darker skin surrounding each nipple.

arrest of labor
A condition in which labor stops progressing, as measured by
cervical dilation.

artificial rupture of membranes (AROM)
A procedure in which your caregiver breaks your bag of waters with an
amnihook (a long plastic device that resembles a crochet needle) in the
attempt to speed up the labor process. Also called *amniotomy*.

asymmetrical
One side of your body is doing something different from the other
side. For example, the lunge, side-lying, and semi-prone positions are
asymmetrical positions.

asynclitic
A position in which your baby's head is tilted and the top of it isn't
centered on the cervix. Can lead to a prolonged labor.

augmentation
Speeding up a slow labor by using self-help methods or interventions such as artificial rupture of membranes (AROM) or Pitocin.

auscultation
Listening to sounds inside your womb, such as your baby's heartbeat. In labor, intermittent auscultation describes how your nurse or caregiver listens to your baby's heartbeat during and between contractions with a Doppler ultrasound stethoscope. At the same time, he or she may place a hand on your abdomen to feel your contractions, then count your baby's heartbeats, noting whether they speed up or slow down and recording the findings.

baby blues
Emotional changes or mood swings that are common in new parents during the first few weeks after the birth of a baby. For example, going from elation to sadness in a matter of minutes isn't uncommon for new parents.

benefit-risk analysis
A process by which your caregiver considers whether treatment will achieve the desired results or create problems, then weighs the treatment's benefits against its risks before forming his or her recommendation for treatment.

beta-endorphins
Your body's natural painkillers, these hormones are secreted when you experience pain, stress, and physical exertion. Also called "endorphins."

birth ball
A large inflatable plastic physical therapy or fitness ball that provides a soft yet firm place to sit comfortably. Used as a comfort tool in labor to enhance mobility and labor progress.

birth doula
Someone (typically a woman) who's trained and experienced in supporting women and their partners during labor and birth.

birth plan
A one- to two-page letter to your caregiver and staff that describes your fears and concerns as well as your wishes and priorities for the treatment of you and your baby. Also called a "birth preference list," "wish list," or "goal sheet."

blastocyst
After conception, the fertilized egg quickly divides from one cell into two, then four, eight, sixteen, and so on until it becomes a multicellular structure called a blastocyst, which begins to implant in your uterus about five to nine days later. Once it's fully implanted, a blastocyst is called an *embryo*.

body mass index (BMI)
A measurement of the relative amounts of fat and muscle in your body. It's calculated by using a ratio of your height to your prepregnancy weight.

Braxton-Hicks contractions
Contractions of the uterine muscle that become more frequent and intense in the third trimester, and that make your uterus hard for about a minute but aren't painful. Unlike labor contractions, Braxton-Hicks contractions don't cause changes in your cervix.

breech presentation
When your baby is positioned with his buttocks, legs, or feet over your cervix, instead of head down (vertex).

castor oil
A strong laxative that causes powerful bowel cramps and contractions, which may initiate uterine contractions to induce labor.

catecholamines
Stress hormones, including epinephrine (adrenaline), norepinephrine, and dopamine. High levels of stress hormones can slow labor progress.

cephalo-pelvic disproportion (CPD)
A condition in which your baby's head is believed to be too large to fit through your pelvis. This diagnosis may be made by your caregiver based on observations during pregnancy, or may be used as a retrospective diagnosis after a prolonged labor that resulted in the birth of a large baby.

certified nurse-midwife (CNM)
A maternity caregiver who has graduated from nursing school, passed an exam to become a registered nurse, and completed one or more years of additional training in midwifery.

certified professional midwife (CPM)
A maternity caregiver who has received training from a variety of sources, including apprenticeship, school, and self-study, and has been the primary attendant at twenty or more births. A CPM practices outside hospitals and provides care similar to that of a licensed midwife.

cervical ripening device
A silicone catheter that's placed within the cervix, then inflated with saline solution. Used to induce labor by accelerating cervical dilation.

cervix
The lower part of the uterus, which protrudes into the vagina.

certified midwives (CMs)
Have graduated from a health-related program other than nursing and must complete the same midwifery training and certification exams that CNMs do. They practice in the same settings as CNMs.

cervical cerclage
When the cervix is closed with suture thread.

cesarean birth
The experience of giving birth by a surgical procedure in which your baby is delivered through incisions in your abdomen and uterus. The procedure is also called a "cesarean section," "C-section," "cesarean delivery," or simply "cesarean."

circumcision
The surgical removal of the foreskin covering the glans (tip) of the penis.

code word
A word that you choose in advance and share with your caregivers. By saying the word during labor, you communicate that, despite your original plan to birth without pain medications, you now want help getting medicated pain relief.

colic
Prolonged crying in a young baby. Typically defined as three or more crying episodes each week for three or more weeks, with each episode lasting three hours or longer.

colostrum
The first breast milk: a highly nutritious yellowish fluid that's low in volume, but high in antibodies and the nutrients your baby will need for the first few days of life before your milk supply increases in volume.

combined spinal-epidural (CSE)
A method for delivering pain medication. CSE uses a spinal narcotic in early labor (which may allow for more mobility), then an epidural anesthetic later in labor, when you need more pain relief.

complicated labor
A labor that is longer, more painful, or more difficult than a normal labor, and may require medical help to ensure the well-being of you and your baby.

conception
Occurs when a sperm fertilizes an egg. The beginning of pregnancy.

contraction
Tightening of the uterine muscle. During labor, these muscle contractions help open your ripe, effaced cervix and help your baby descend. Contractions become more frequent and more intense as labor progresses.

corticosteroids
Medications that may be given to speed up the maturation of your baby's lungs if a preterm birth can't be prevented.

corticotropin-releasing hormone (CRH)
Comes from your baby, the placenta, and tissues within your uterus. Increased levels of CRH in late pregnancy may help initiate labor.

crowning
The third phase of the second stage of labor. It begins when the widest part of your baby's head is visible at the vaginal opening and no longer retreats between pushes, and it ends with her birth.

delayed pushing
An option for the second stage of labor, in which a woman who doesn't have an urge to push (such as after receiving an epidural) may wait an hour or two, or until her baby's head crowns, before pushing actively. Also called *passive descent*.

descent
The downward movement of your baby into your pelvis.

diagnostic test
Term used to describe a test that is more specific and more reliable than a screening test in identifying a woman with a pregnancy complication or a baby with a problem.

dilation
The opening of the cervix, which allows your baby to pass through for birth.

directed pushing
An option for the second stage of labor, in which your caregiver tells you how long and how hard to push. This method is used if you can't feel your contractions and delayed pushing isn't an option or if spontaneous pushing isn't effective.

Doppler ultrasound
A device that uses sound waves to monitor your baby's heart rate. Typically used at prenatal visits as well as during labor and birth.

due date
An estimate of when your baby will be born. The majority of babies are born in the period from two weeks before their due dates to two weeks after their due dates.

early labor
Usually the longest phase of the first stage of labor, often because contractions are further apart, shorter, and less intense than they'll be later in labor. Contractions are generally more than five minutes apart, and you can walk and talk during them. Also called the *latent phase*.

ectopic
An ectopic pregnancy occurs when the fertilized egg implants itself outside the uterus, usually in the wall of a fallopian tube (called a tubal pregnancy) but sometimes in the cervix, ovary, or abdomen. Most ectopic pregnancies can't develop into a live birth and typically require medical intervention to manage.

effacement
The thinning and shortening of the cervix in preparation for birth.

elective induction
An induction done without a medical reason, either because a woman requested induction or because her caregiver recommended it. Also called a "social induction."

electronic fetal monitoring (EFM)
Used to monitor your baby's heart rate and your contractions, to assess how your baby is responding to labor. There are two types of EFM. External EFM uses belts to hold two sensors on your abdomen, and the less commonly used internal EFM uses two sensors placed inside your uterus.

embryo
By two weeks after conception, your baby is called an embryo.

engagement
About two weeks before the birth, your baby descends deeper into your pelvis. You may feel less pressure on your diaphragm and find breathing and eating easier. Also called *lightening* or "dropping."

engorgement
Painful swelling of the breasts.

epidural catheter
A tube inserted into the epidural space near the spinal nerves and used to deliver pain medication.

episiotomy
A surgical incision of the perineum that enlarges the vaginal outlet. Once common practice, now the majority of caregivers use it only when medically necessary to deliver the baby quickly.

estrogen
A hormone that promotes the growth of the uterine muscles and their blood supply, encourages production of vaginal mucus, and stimulates the development of the ductal system and blood supply in the breasts. In late pregnancy, rising estrogen levels increase the uterus's sensitivity to oxytocin and help start labor.

evert
To draw out your nipple to allow your baby to latch on well for nursing. Typically occurs when your baby suckles.

expression
Removing milk from the breast by hand or by using a pump. May be used to relieve fullness, maintain milk supply, or store milk for your baby's consumption.

expulsion breathing
A way to breathe during spontaneous bearing down. During the pushing stage, use relaxed breathing when you don't have the urge to push. When you have an urge to push, you may briefly hold your breath and bear down, or you may exhale with an open throat while pushing.

external version
A procedure used to attempt to manually turn a baby from a breech or transverse position to a head-down position (vertex).

failure to progress
Term used either to describe a labor that's taking longer than expected for the cervix to dilate to 10 centimeters, or to describe a pushing stage that's taking longer than expected. May be treated with augmentation or cesarean delivery; however, if your baby is handling labor well, you may also ask whether self-help measures can effectively help with labor progress.

fallopian tubes
Provide the path for an egg to travel from your ovaries to your uterus.

false positives
Describes situations in which test results for a condition are positive, but the condition isn't present (for example, the fetal heart rate pattern indicates distress, but your baby turns out to be fine).

family physician
A physician who has graduated from medical school or a school of osteopathic medicine and has completed two or more years of additional training in family medicine, including maternity and pediatric care.

feeding cues
How your baby shows he's hungry. Include rooting, mouthing, tongue thrusts, sucking, and increased activity levels. Crying is a late feeding cue, used when the other cues have gone unnoticed.

fetal intolerance of labor
See *abnormal fetal heart rate*. Also called "fetal distress."

first stage of labor
The period that begins when contractions are becoming longer, stronger, and closer together (progressing) and ends when your cervix is completely dilated.

forceps
A tool (steel tongs) that's used to assist with a vaginal birth.

foremilk
Breast milk produced early in the feeding. Foremilk is lower in fat and higher in sugar than hindmilk.

fourth stage of labor
Begins after the placenta is delivered and ends one to several hours later, when your and your baby's conditions have stabilized.

freestanding birth center
A birth center unaffiliated with a hospital.

fundus
The top of your uterus.

general anesthesia
A systemic medication that causes a total loss of sensation and consciousness.

gestation
Another term for pregnancy, which lasts an average of 280 days or forty weeks after the first day of your last menstrual period.

gestational age
The age of your baby from the first day of your last menstrual period. Note that conception occurs within twelve to twenty-four hours after ovulation, which typically occurs fourteen days after the beginning of your last period. So, two weeks after conception your baby's gestational age is four weeks.

gestational hypertension
High blood pressure that develops during pregnancy, defined as at least two consecutive readings that are over 140/90. This condition affects 10 percent of pregnant women in the United States. Also called *pregnancy-induced hypertension (PIH)*.

glycemic index
An index that ranks foods according to how quickly and significantly they elevate your blood sugar.

Group B streptococcus (GBS)
A type of bacteria. If you test positive for GBS in pregnancy, you may be given antibiotics during labor.

hemorrhoids
Swollen varicose veins in the rectal area that may be as small as a pea or as large as a grape.

Heparin Lock
Involves inserting an intravenous (IV) catheter, but doesn't require hooking it to an IV bag and pole until IV fluids are needed. Also called "Hep-Lock."

hindmilk
Breast milk produced later in a feeding session, released with the let-down reflex. This milk provides most of the calories and contains more fat and protein than foremilk.

homeopathy
A complementary medicine technique that uses diluted derivatives of natural substances to stimulate your body to respond in a way that heals or corrects a specific problem, such as a labor that won't start.

human chorionic gonadotropin (hCG)
A hormone produced only during pregnancy. It ensures that your ovaries produce estrogen and progesterone for the first two to three months of your pregnancy, until your placenta matures and produces the appropriate amount.

hyperventilation
Overbreathing. If you find yourself feeling lightheaded or dizzy while using a breathing technique, try either slowing down your breathing, focusing on the exhalation rather than the inhalation, or breathing into your cupped hands.

immunization
See *vaccination*.

incompetent cervix
A cervix that shortens and opens in midpregnancy without preterm labor contractions.

incontinence
A condition that causes you to leak urine when you have a full bladder, exercise, cough, or sneeze (urinary incontinence) or uncontrollably pass gas or leak stool (fecal incontinence).

induction
An intervention used to start labor.

infant cues
Your baby's nonverbal communication. For example, when she's over-stimulated, she may close his eyes, yawn, get glassy—eyed, turn away, or stiffen. If you miss these cues and continue to stimulate her, she may begin a prolonged bout of crying.

informed choice
See *informed decision*.

informed consent
After becoming informed about an option or treatment, you agree to it.

informed decision
The decision you make to refuse or consent to a health care option or medical treatment, after becoming informed about it through research and consultation with your caregiver and other knowledgeable medical professionals, as well as with supportive friends and family. Also called *informed choice*.

informed refusal
After becoming informed about an option or treatment, you refuse it.

inhalation medication
A gas you breathe to receive pain medication.

intervention
A medical procedure used to intervene in the natural labor process, such as induction, augmentation, episiotomy, or cesarean surgery.

intramuscular (IM) medication
A shot given into a muscle to deliver medication.

intrathecal space
The space inside the dura (the membrane that surrounds your spinal cord) that's filled with cerebrospinal fluid. It's where spinal medications are injected.

intravenous (IV) catheter
A tube that's inserted into a vein through a needle, allowing fluids and medications to be given directly into your circulatory system.

intravenous (IV) medication
An injection into a vein, often through an IV catheter, to deliver medication.

involution
After the birth, your uterus begins the six-week process of contracting to its nonpregnant size.

jaundice
An excess of bilirubin that causes your baby's skin or the whites of his eyes to become yellow by the third or fourth day after the birth.

Kegel
An exercise used to maintain the tone of your pelvic floor muscles, improve blood circulation in that area, decrease the incidence and severity of hemorrhoids and incontinence, and support your uterus and other pelvic organs.

lactation consultant
A breastfeeding expert.

lanugo
Fine, downy hair that develops on your baby's arms, legs, and back while in the womb.

latch
Your baby's connection with the breast to feed. A good latch permits your baby to nurse effectively.

latent phase
See *early labor*.

lay midwife
A maternity caregiver who might or might not be legally registered with the state or province, and whose qualifications and standards of care might or might not meet state or provincial standards. Also called "empirical midwife."

Leopold's maneuvers
The technique your caregiver uses to determine the baby's position by feeling your abdomen.

let-down reflex
When your baby nurses, the suckling stimulates your pituitary gland to release oxytocin, which makes your milk-producing cells contract and release (let down) milk for your baby to drink.

leukorrhea
A thin, liquid mucus discharge from the vagina.

licensed midwife (LM)
A maternity caregiver who has completed up to three years of formal midwifery training according to state requirements.

lightening
See *engagement*.

local anesthetic
Injection or application of pain medication that affects a specific, relatively small part of your body.

lochia
The heavy red discharge that flows from your vagina in the six weeks after the birth. It's made of the extra blood and fluid that supported your pregnancy and the uterine lining that sustained your baby.

malposition
When your baby is in an unfavorable position in the womb, which may lead to a prolonged labor. Can often be corrected by changing positions frequently.

mastitis
An infection of the breast.

meconium
Your baby's first bowel movements, a collection of digestive enzymes and residue from swallowed amniotic fluid. Appears as a sticky, greenish-black substance.

membranes
The amnion and chorion membranes create the amniotic sac that surrounds your baby in your uterus.

miscarriage
The unexpected death and delivery of a baby before the twentieth week of pregnancy. Also called "spontaneous abortion."

misoprostol (Cytotec)
A medication used to induce labor.

Montgomery glands
Small bumps on your areolae that secrete a lubricating substance that keeps the nipple supple and prevents infection.

morning sickness
Nausea and vomiting in the early months of pregnancy. Despite its name, morning sickness can occur at any time of day.

moxibustion
A version of acupuncture that doesn't use needles but instead uses burning herbs placed close to the acupuncture points.

mucous plug
Mucus that fills the cervical opening during pregnancy to provide a barrier to help protect your baby.

multipara
A woman who has given birth more than once.

multiples
Two or more babies gestating in the same womb.

narcotics and narcotic-like drugs
Medications that reduce the transmission of pain messages to the pain receptors in your brain.

naturopathic doctor (ND)
A health care provider who has completed three to four years of post-graduate training in natural medicine. May also have taken an additional year of midwifery training to be able to provide prenatal care and attend births.

neonatal intensive care unit (NICU)
A hospital unit where medically challenged newborns stay for monitoring and treatment until they can breathe on their own, stay warm at room temperature, and breastfeed or take a bottle.

neuraxial medications
Drugs that are injected into the space surrounding the spinal cord (neuraxis), such as epidurals and spinal blocks.

nipple confusion
A condition experienced by some babies who have difficulty adapting to different sucking patterns and flows of liquid, when they're fed alternately by a bottle and at the breast.

nullipara
A woman who has never given birth.

obstetrician/gynecologist (OB-GYN)
A physician who has graduated from medical school or a school of osteopathic medicine and has had three or more years of additional training in obstetrics and gynecology.

occiput anterior
The back of baby's head (occiput) is toward the front of your body.

occiput posterior
The back of baby's head (occiput) is toward your back.

occiput transverse (ROT or LOT)
The back of your baby's head is toward your right (or left) side.

oral medication
A pill or liquid you swallow to receive a medication.

ovaries
Female sex glands where eggs are produced.

ovulation
When a ripened egg is released into your fallopian tubes. On average, this happens fourteen days after the first day of your last menstrual period. If you have intercourse between four days before and one day after ovulation, there's a chance of conception.

ovum
An egg produced by a woman. When an egg is fertilized by a sperm, conception occurs.

oxytocin
A hormone produced in your pituitary gland, which stimulates uterine contractions to help trigger the onset of labor and promote labor progress. Also present during orgasm and during breastfeeding, it's often called "the love hormone."

pain modifiers
External stimuli that affect your awareness and perception of pain.

parity
Describes the condition of having given birth.

passive descent
See *delayed pushing*.

patient-controlled epidural analgesia (PCEA)
A device that allows you to increase your epidural dosage when you need more pain relief.

pediatric and family nurse practitioner
A registered nurse who has additional training in pediatrics or family health. Provides well-child care and treats common illnesses.

pediatrician
A physician who specializes in children's health care.

pelvic floor muscles
Muscles attached to the pelvis that support your abdominal and pelvic organs. These muscles form a figure-eight around your urethra, vagina, and anus.

perinatologist
An obstetrician/gynecologist (OB-GYN) who has received further training and certification in managing very high-risk pregnancies and births.

perineal massage
A massage that stretches the inner tissue of your lower vagina. Can be used during pregnancy or the second stage of labor to relax the tissue so it will stretch around your baby's head.

perineum
The external genitals (labia, urethra, clitoris, vaginal opening) and anus.

phototherapy
A medical procedure used to treat jaundice that shines a special type of cool light on your baby's skin, causing the bilirubin level to drop.

Pitocin
Commonly referred to as "Pit," this is a synthetic version of oxytocin.

placenta
An organ that develops in pregnancy, the placenta produces hormones and exchanges oxygen, nutrients, and waste products for your developing baby. It's released and delivered shortly after your baby's birth.

position
Refers to where the back of your baby's head (occiput) is in relation to your body.

positive signs of labor
Include contractions that become longer, stronger, and more frequent (progressing) and the rupture of membranes in a gush of amniotic fluid. These are the only reliable signs that labor has begun and your cervix is dilating.

possible signs of labor
Occur in late pregnancy and may indicate that hormonal changes are underway but cervical changes aren't yet occurring. These signs occur intermittently for days or weeks, but they don't indicate labor.

post-date pregnancy
A pregnancy that has lasted to at least forty-two weeks. Although the average length of pregnancy is forty weeks, many pregnancies last longer. Caregivers may misuse the term "post-date" as early as forty weeks.

postmaturity
A condition in which the placenta stops functioning well, the baby's growth slows or stops, and the risk of stillbirth increases. True postmaturity is rare even in babies born two weeks after their due dates. "Postmature babies" at birth have an absence of lanugo, scant vernix caseosa; long fingernails and toenails; and dry, peeling, or cracked skin.

postpartum depression
A condition that generally presents itself between two weeks to one year after the birth. Symptoms vary in severity among women.

postpartum doula
Someone (typically a woman) who's trained and experienced with helping a woman and her family adjust to postpartum life by teaching them about newborns' needs and abilities, and about infant feeding, sleep, and cues, while providing assistance with household tasks.

postpartum hemorrhage
The excessive loss of blood (more than 500 milliliters or 2 cups) during the first twenty-four hours after the birth.

postpartum mood disorders (PPMD)
Emotional conditions that can develop in the first year after birth, such as anxiety and panic disorder, obsessive-compulsive disorder, postpartum depression, bipolar disorder, and post-traumatic stress disorder.

postpartum psychosis
A rare condition that occurs in women after the birth and requires immediate care and psychiatric treatment. Symptoms include severe agitation, mood swings, depression, and delusions.

precipitate birth
A birth that results from a very fast labor. For a first-time mother, may be defined as an entire labor that lasts six hours or less, but it's more often applied to a labor that is three hours or less. For a woman who has previously given birth, it's one hour or less.

preeclampsia
High blood pressure and protein in the urine. A multi-organ condition with mild to severe symptoms that affects 5 to 8 percent of pregnancies. Previously called "toxemia."

pregnancy-induced hypertension (PIH)
See *gestational hypertension*.

prelabor signs of labor
Indicate that your cervix is probably moving forward, ripening, or effacing. These signs may progress into positive labor signs the same day they begin, or they may simply alert you that labor will begin in a few days or weeks.

prelabor
A period of hours or days in which you experience contractions, but your cervix isn't actively dilating. It's likely that these contractions are getting your cervix ready to dilate by moving it forward and helping it ripen and efface. Prelabor contractions may range from as little as thirty seconds long and twenty minutes apart, to as much as one or two minutes long and five to eight minutes apart. However, the contractions change very little in length, frequency, and intensity over time (nonprogressing).

premature
A baby that's born before the thirty-seventh week of pregnancy.

presentation
Describes the part of your baby that's lying over your cervix and will emerge from your body first. Also called *presenting part*.

presenting part
See *presentation*.

preterm labor
A labor that begins before the thirty-seventh week of pregnancy.

primigravida
A woman who is pregnant for the first time.

primipara
A woman who has given birth once.

progesterone
A hormone that relaxes your uterus during pregnancy, keeping it from contracting too much. It also relaxes the walls of blood vessels (helping you maintain a healthy blood pressure) and the walls of your stomach and bowels (allowing for greater absorption of nutrients).

progressing contractions
Contractions that become longer, stronger, and more frequent over time.

prolactin
A hormone that's produced after the birth and stimulates the production of breast milk.

prolapsed cord
A rare condition that occurs when the water breaks and the umbilical cord slips below the baby so it's either in the vagina or lying between the baby and the cervix. Requires a call to 911 and transport to the hospital for an immediate cesarean.

prolonged labor
A labor that progresses more slowly than expected. Diagnosis is somewhat subjective.

prolonged prelabor
Prelabor that lasts longer than a day.

prostaglandin
A hormone produced in your amniotic membrane. Increased levels in late pregnancy ripen your cervix in preparation for labor and stimulate muscles in your uterus and bowels to begin labor.

quickening
Describes the moment when you feel your baby's movements for the first time, during the second trimester.

regional anesthetic
Pain medication that affects a large area of your body.

relaxin
A hormone from your ovaries that relaxes and softens your ligaments, cartilage, and cervix, making these tissues more stretchable during pregnancy and letting your pelvic joints spread during birth.

respiratory distress syndrome (RDS)
A condition in which a newborn infant has difficulty breathing and is unable to get sufficient oxygen due to immature lungs. The most common complication of premature birth, it requires immediate medical treatment.

rhythm
Women who cope well in labor rely on rhythm in various forms. Rhythmic activity calms the mind and lets a woman work well with her body.

ripening
The softening of the cervix.

ritual
The repetition of a meaningful rhythmic activity during contractions to increase your ability to cope.

routine
Procedures or treatment that's offered to all pregnant women and their newborns, regardless of medical status.

rupture of membranes
Breaking of the bag of waters that may manifest itself either as the leaking of a small amount of amniotic fluid from the vagina, or as a gush of fluids. Rupture may happen before labor or may signal the onset of labor, or it can happen at any point during labor and birth.

screening test
A medical test that can rule out a particular condition or may indicate an increased chance that the condition is present. In the latter case, a diagnostic test confirms the condition.

second stage of labor
The birth of your baby. This stage begins when your cervix is fully dilated and ends when your baby is born.

serial induction
Medication to induce labor is given during the day, but is discontinued at night to allow you to eat and sleep.

shared decision making
A collaborative approach to making an informed decision, in which you and your caregiver discuss the medical risks and benefits of treatment and any possible alternatives.

special care nursery
A hospital unit for newborns who need extra medical monitoring or support, but don't need the intensive care of a NICU.

spinal block
An injection of anesthetic near the spinal nerves that takes effect quickly and lasts for an hour or two.

spit up
When a baby expels a dribble or more of milk (up to 2 to 3 tablespoons is common) after a feeding.

spontaneous bearing down
An option for the second stage of labor, in which you naturally bear down or strain for five to six seconds at a time and take several breaths between efforts. This type of pushing makes more oxygen available to your baby than if you hold your breath and bear down for as long as possible.

spontaneous rituals
Methods of coping invented by you over the course of your labor and reinforced by your support team. May include positions, movement, repeated words or sounds, specific kinds of touch, and so on.

station
Refers to the location of the top of your baby's head (or other presenting part) within your pelvis. Descent is measured by station.

sterile water block
An alternative option for relief of back pain during labor. A caregiver or nurse injects tiny amounts of sterile water into four places on your lower back. The injections cause severe stinging for a minute or more, but then provide pain relief by rapidly increasing endorphin production.

sudden infant death syndrome (SIDS)
The sudden death of a baby younger than one year that remains unexplained after a thorough investigation. There are steps that can be taken to further reduce the rare chance of SIDS; however, for about 1 in 2,000 babies, it appears to be impossible to predict or prevent.

supine hypotension
When lying on your back makes your uterus press on the abdominal vein that carries blood from your legs to your heart (inferior vena cava), causing a drop in blood pressure.

surfactant
A substance that allows your baby's lungs to expand during an inhalation and remain partially inflated during an exhalation.

synthetic prostaglandins
Medications that mimic the hormone prostaglandin.

systemic
Describes a medication that affects your entire body.

tandem nursing
Breastfeeding two children at the same time (such as twins or your baby and toddler).

tension spots
Body areas that you habitually tense when stressed. For example, your shoulders, forehead, mouth, jaw, or fists.

third stage of labor
Begins with the birth of your baby and ends with the delivery of the placenta.

Three Rs: relaxation, rhythm, and ritual
A theory about how women cope with labor when given support and freedom to explore coping options. You stay as relaxed as possible throughout labor, until you discover your coping rhythm. Your partner's role is to reinforce this ritual for as long as it continues to help you.

tocolytic medication
A drug used to slow or stop contractions; for example, during preterm labor.

transition
Final phase of the first stage of labor, which serves as the transition to the second stage of labor. Your cervix is reaching complete dilation, and your baby is beginning to descend into your birth canal. Contractions are ninety seconds to two minutes long and two to three minutes apart.

transverse incision
The most common incision (cut) for a cesarean birth. Horizontal incision on the lower abdomen (at the "bikini line") through the bottom of the uterus.

transverse lie
When your baby is positioned sideways in the uterus, with his back or shoulder closest to the cervix. Only occurs in 1 in 2,500 births. Your caregiver will attempt an external version to turn your baby, and if unsuccessful, your baby will be delivered by cesarean.

triage
Observation area in the hospital, where an admitting nurse assesses your condition, your pattern of contractions, your dilation (with a vaginal exam), and your baby's well-being, in order to determine whether you're ready to be admitted to the hospital, or whether you should return home with instructions on when to return.

trial of labor after cesarean (TOLAC)
When a woman with a prior cesarean chooses to let labor begin and progress, with the hope of having a vaginal birth after cesarean (VBAC).

trimesters
Pregnancy is divided into three trimesters, each one lasting about three months.

ultrasound
See *Doppler ultrasound and ultrasound scan*.

ultrasound scan
Equipment that uses intermittent transmission of sound waves to help your caregiver "see" inside the uterus. Can be used as a screening test or a diagnostic test for evaluating your baby's development.

umbilical cord
Links the placenta to your baby's navel, and together the umbilical cord and placenta pass oxygen and nutrients from you to your baby. While the placenta provides a barrier against most (but not all) bacteria in your bloodstream, most viruses and drugs cross to your baby. The placenta also exchanges waste products from your baby, which your blood then carries to your kidneys and lungs for excretion.

urge to push
The most significant sign of the second stage of labor. You may find yourself holding your breath and straining or grunting during each contraction.

uterine atony
Poor uterine muscle tone. The most frequent cause of postpartum hemorrhage.

uterine rupture
The separation of a uterine incision from a previous cesarean or uterine surgery.

uterus
A hollow, muscular organ the size and shape of a pear in which a baby develops.

vaccination
An administration of a vaccine to prevent illness. Also called *immunization*.

vacuum extractor
A tool (silicone suction cup) that's used to assist with a vaginal delivery.

vaginal birth after cesarean (VBAC)
A vaginal birth after a previous cesarean, as a result of a successful trial of labor after cesarean (TOLAC).

vernix caseosa
A white, creamy substance that protected your baby's skin in your womb.

vertex
Presentation in which the top of your baby's head is down over your cervix.

wireless (or telemetry) monitoring
Wireless electronic fetal monitoring, which allows you to walk and use the shower or bath.

Index

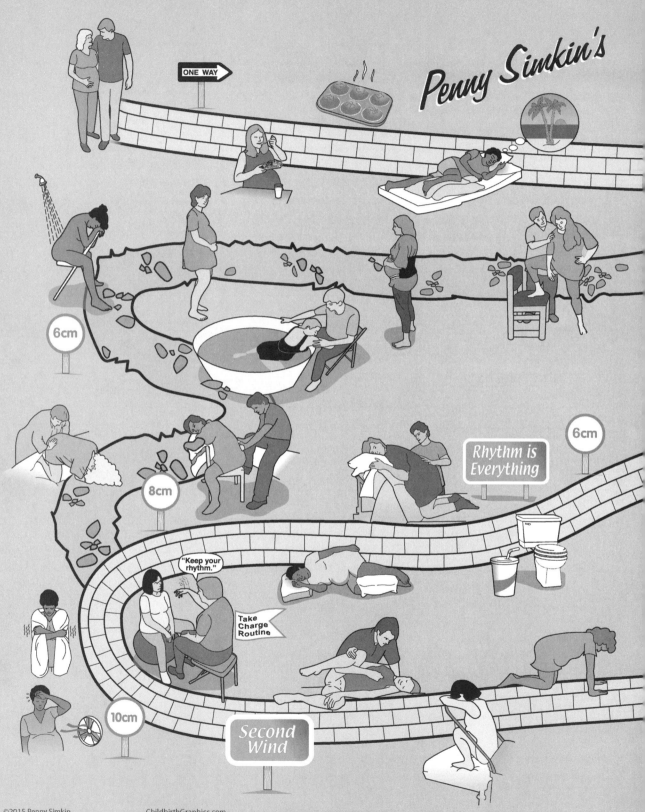

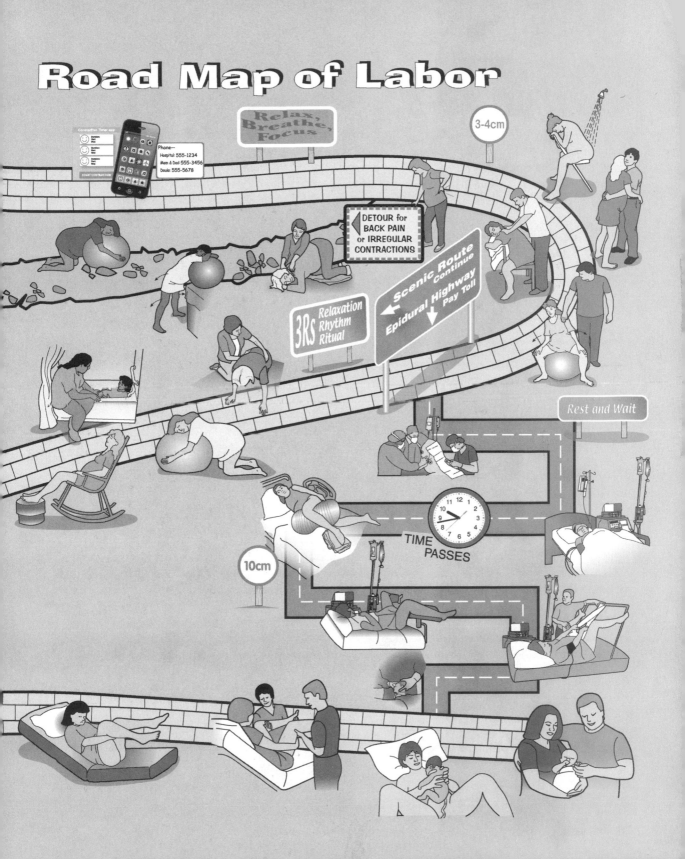

Also from Meadowbrook Press

100,000 Baby Names

From the #1 baby name book author, this is the most complete guide for helping you name your baby. It contains more than 100,000 popular and unusual names from around the world, complete with origins, meanings, variations, and famous namesakes. It also includes the most recently available top 100 names for girls and boys, as well as over 600 helpful lists of names to consider and avoid.

Pregnancy, Childbirth, and the Newborn

More complete and up-to-date than any other pregnancy guide, this remarkable book is the "bible" for childbirth educators. Now revised with a greatly expanded treatment of pregnancy tests, complications, and infections; an expanded list of drugs and medications (plus advice for uses); and a brand-new chapter on creating a detailed birth plan.

First-Year Baby Care

This is one of the leading baby-care books to guide you through your baby's first year. It contains step-by-step information on the basics of baby care, including bathing, diapering, medical facts, and feeding your baby.

Baby & Child Emergency First Aid

Edited by Mitchell J. Einzig, MD and Paula Kelly, MD. This user-friendly book is the next best thing to 911, with a quick-reference index, large illustrations, and easy-to-read instructions on handling the most common childhood emergencies.

Baby Play & Learn

Child-development expert Penny Warner offers 160 ideas for games and activities that provide hours of developmental learning opportunities. It includes bulleted lists of skills baby learns through play, step-by-step instructions for each game and activity, and illustrations that demonstrate how to play many of the games.

Feed Me! I'm Yours

This is easy-to-use, economical guide to making baby food at home. More than 200 recipes cover everything a parent needs to know about teething foods, nutritious snacks, and quick, pleasing lunches.

We offer many more titles written to delight, inform, and entertain.
To browse our full selection of titles, visit our website at:

www.MeadowbrookPress.com

For quantity discounts, please call: 1-800-338-2232
Meadowbrook Press • 6110 Blue Circle Drive, Suite 237 • Minnetonka, MN • 55343